SERIES OF STUDIES IN
TUDOR AND STUART LITERATURE

General Editors

F. H. MARES *and* A. T. BRISSENDEN

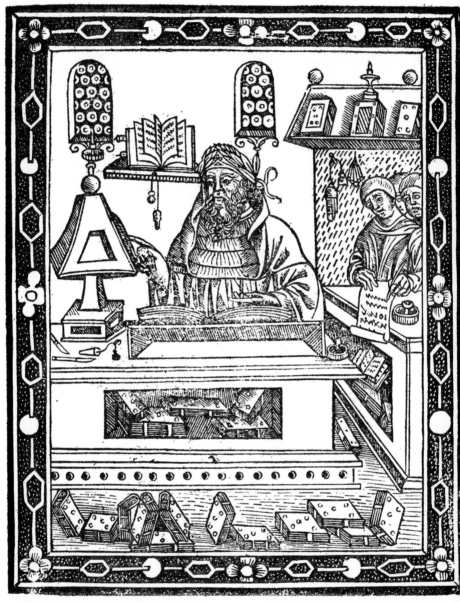

Albertus Magnus studies while his students take notes. *The Book of Secrets* was probably compiled by one such student; in this picture he would most appropriately be represented by the student in the middle of the three.

From *Liber Secretorum Alberti Magni* (1502)

THE BOOK OF SECRETS
OF ALBERTUS MAGNUS

of the Virtues of Herbs, Stones
and Certain Beasts

ALSO

A BOOK OF THE MARVELS
OF THE WORLD

Edited by

MICHAEL R. BEST

and

FRANK H. BRIGHTMAN

OXFORD
AT THE CLARENDON PRESS
1973

Oxford University Press, Ely House, London W. 1

GLASGOW NEW YORK TORONTO MELBOURNE WELLINGTON
CAPE TOWN IBADAN NAIROBI DAR ES SALAAM LUSAKA ADDIS ABABA
DELHI BOMBAY CALCUTTA MADRAS KARACHI LAHORE DACCA
KUALA LUMPUR SINGAPORE HONG KONG TOKYO

*Printed in Great Britain
at the University Press, Oxford
by Vivian Ridler
Printer to the University*

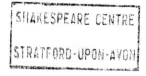

ACKNOWLEDGEMENTS

IN the section of *The Book of Secrets* which deals with the properties of stones, we are indebted to the research of Dorothy Wyckoff in her translation of Albertus Magnus's *Mineralia* (*Book of Minerals*, Oxford, 1967). We would like to thank the General Editors for their guidance and encouragement, and Dr. H. H. Huxley for his help on problems with the medieval Latin text.

M. R. B.

F. H. B.

PREFACE

THIS is the second volume in the series of Studies in Tudor and Stuart Literature, the aim of which is to make available a number of works of the sixteenth and seventeenth centuries which are of interest for their literary or historic value, or as documents in the history of taste and culture. The texts are established from the examination of early editions and manuscripts, taking into account the work of previous editors where necessary. The introduction sets the work in its social and literary context, discussing the author in his time, the work itself, and the treatment of the text. Annotations are intended to elucidate difficult passages, discuss usage, comment on textual problems, and refer the reader to other editions and relevant material.

The research leading to this publication has been supported by the Australian Research Grants Committee, and, as general editors, we gratefully acknowledge this assistance. We are also happy to thank Miss Robin Eaden and Mr. Patrick Greenland for their help in checking information and proofs.

F. H. MARES
A. T. BRISSENDEN

Department of English
University of Adelaide

CONTENTS

LIST OF ILLUSTRATIONS

INTRODUCTION

1. The Nature and Origin of *The Book of Secrets*

The Book of Secrets was one of the most widely known works in a literature which gained great popularity during the Middle Ages. There were many books of 'secrets' dealing with the marvellous properties, real or imagined, of beasts, herbs, stones, and the human body; there were books of anecdotes, usually associated with a famous name like Alexander the Great, and there were even more which, like *The Book of Secrets*, collected their material from all these sources. The popularity of these works is demonstrated by the survival of a great many manuscripts from as early as the twelfth century and by the fact that several continued to be copied, anthologized, translated, and printed well into the seventeenth century.[1]

The literature of secrets was in another sense a popular tradition; at no time did scholars of repute contribute to it, and indeed they seldom commented on books of this kind at all, except perhaps to attack them. The Italian humanist, Pico della Mirandola (1463-94), writing about what was probably one of the sources of *The Book of Secrets*, remarked unflatteringly that it was 'stuffed with execrable dreams and figments'.[2] Despite the scorn of the scholars, however, the popular literaʹ ture capitalized on the prestige associated with the great scholars of the past; Aristotle, Plato, Galen, and (in the case of the present work) Albertus Magnus had many works spuriously attributed to them. This is scarcely surprising when we realize

---

[1] For an extensive discussion of this literature, see Lynn Thorndike's *History of Magic and Experimental Science* (New York, 1923), vol. ii. A brief summary will be found on pp. xxxix ff. below.

[2] *Disputationes Adversus Astrologiam*, i, quoted by Thorndike, ii. 779.

that the intellectual climate of the time was such that original thinkers like Albertus Magnus felt constrained to cast their writings in the form of commentaries on the works of the ancients; the whole of Albertus's considerable output was in⁄ tended by the author to be a commentary on Aristotle, though it contains much original thought. Lesser writers accepted the same convention with fewer scruples.

The most interesting thing about *The Book of Secrets* is not that it was written, but that its popularity continued so long. The present text is taken from the first English edition, printed in about 1550, but the last edition did not appear until almost ninety years later, in 1637; since there were seven known editions between these two, *The Book of Secrets* retained a steady interest throughout the Elizabethan and early Stuart periods. It is the aim of this introduction, and of the present edition as a whole, to examine the attitudes towards the 'marvellous' of that section of the Elizabethan public which continued to read *The Book of Secrets*.

As its Latin name, *Liber aggregationis*, or 'book of collected items', suggests, *The Book of Secrets* is an anthology rather than a single work. It is divided initially into sections dealing with the marvellous properties of herbs, stones, and beasts; there is a brief treatise on astrology, and there is what originally was a different book, a collection of the 'marvels of the world'. Even within these various sections, however, there are parts collected from widely differing sources; the section on herbs, for example, is divided into two parts, sixteen herbs with their magical properties in the first part, and seven herbs with their astrological and medical properties in the second. Some of the sub⁄sections of the work, and some of the individual magic recipes, can be traced to some kind of 'source', but for the most part this tells us little about the origin of the work, since the source itself is an anthology from largely untraced sources.

As an anthology, *The Book of Secrets* can be divided into its component parts; where these sections fit into the pattern of European thought will be discussed later.

1. *On Herbs:*

(*a*) There are sixteen herbs described in terms of their magical properties. The nature of the recipes, and the fact that the names of the plants are given (supposedly) in Greek and Aramaic, suggest that these are taken from the same source as the 'beasts' below.

(*b*) There are seven herbs 'after the mind of Alexander' which are dealt with primarily in terms of astrological and medical properties. They are taken from a work ascribed to one Alexius Affricus or Flaccus Africanus, rather than, as the text suggests, Alexander the Great.[3]

2. *On Stones:*

(*a*) A total of forty-five entries are taken from the lapidary of Albertus Magnus.

(*b*) This is followed by a single, rather confused paragraph, supposedly taken from Isidore of Seville, the seventh-century encyclopedist.

3. *On Beasts:*

(*a*) There are eighteen beasts—animals, birds, and fishes—probably taken from the same source as the first group of herbs.

(*b*) Again there is a short section, supposedly from Isidore.

4. *On the Astrological Influence of the Planets:*

(*a*) Originally there was a treatise on the hours of the day governed by the various planets, followed by a very brief discussion of the qualities of the planets.

(*b*) In later English editions a fuller treatment of the astrological qualities of the planets was included.

5. *On the Marvels of the World:*

(*a*) The Latin text began with a theoretical discussion of magic (assuming its efficacy) followed by a further discussion

---

[3] Thorndike, ii. 233, 728.

establishing the necessity for experiment rather than theorizing in natural science. The Elizabethan translator omitted the references to magic.

(b) There follow a large number of random recipes from various sources. This section may have been taken from a similar anthology, the *Liber Vaccae*, or *Liber Auguemis*, attributed variously to Galen or Plato.[4]

(c) The recipes change abruptly in nature and format (many of them conjuring tricks, or supposedly hallucinogenic suffumigations). This final section appears to have come from the *Book of Fires* by Marcus Grecus.[5]

There is not much we can gather about the compiler of the text, the 'author', from this list. It is tempting to think that he added the short sections 'from Isidore', and perhaps the treatise on the hours of the planets, for this would leave five probable sources, supplemented by his own gleanings in 'marvels'. Certainly it was the marvellous, or sensational, which interested him; we see this throughout in the whole tone of the work, of course, but most interestingly in the one section taken from a reliable source, the 'stones' from the lapidary of Albertus Magnus. The lapidary was originally part of a much larger work, the *Mineralia*, in which Albertus attempted to organize the known theory and knowledge of minerals. Albertus seems to have believed in the powers of the stones he listed; one section of the *Mineralia* (ii. 1. 1) is a defence of the concept that stones had what we would now call magical powers, referring, as does the writer of the *Marvels of the World*, to the undoubted power of the magnet as a justification for belief in more re-markable properties in other stones. No such philosophical discussion is attempted in *The Book of Secrets*, however; even when individual stones are being considered, the compiler

---

[4] Thorndike, ii. 777 ff.

[5] Thorndike, ii. 738; the Latin text of the *Book of Fires* is published with a parallel French translation in Pierre E. M. Berthelot's *La Chimie au moyen âge* (Paris, 1893), vol. i.

tends to omit the passages in Albertus Magnus which are in any way sceptical. The passage on the 'eagle stone' *Aetites* (or *Echites*) in *The Book of Secrets*, for example, omits a great deal of interesting comment by Albertus Magnus on the habits of cranes, which, he has observed, take stones into their nests, but do not seem to be very particular about which stone they use. See also the note on *liparea* (p. 42).

The compiler of the text associated *The Book of Secrets* more firmly with Albertus Magnus than by merely borrowing one section of the book from him. Both the preface and a passage at the end of the section on beasts attribute the work to Albertus, and there has been serious discussion as to whether the whole book is in fact by him.[6] It should be clear that the intellectual tenor of *The Book of Secrets* is very different from the known works of Albertus Magnus, and yet it is also clear that it was written at a time either contemporary with Albertus, or very soon after his death; the earliest manuscripts surviving are from the late thirteenth century,[7] and Albertus died in 1279. It may be that *The Book of Secrets* was written by a follower of Albertus; certainly, as Thorndike says, 'There can be little doubt that it pretends to be a product of his experimental school among the Dominicans at Cologne' (vol. ii, p. 730).

The scholarly pretension of *The Book of Secrets* is not limited to its attribution to Albertus Magnus. The sections on herbs and on beasts both claim to give the names of the plants or animals in Greek or Chaldean (Aramaic); however, the names given seem to have no relation to the languages they are supposedly derived from.[8] Either the names were made up by the original writer, in order to impress the reader, or textual corruption of the unfamiliar words has been so extreme that they have become nonsense. The second possibility is not as

[6] Thorndike, ii. 738; see also his article, 'Further Consideration of the *Experimenta*, *Speculum Astronomiae* and *De Secretis Mulierum* Ascribed to Albertus Magnus', *Speculum*, xxx (1955), 413-33.

[7] Thorndike, *History*, ii. 271 ff.

[8] Thorndike, 'Further Consideration of the *Experimenta* . . .'; see also the note on *Magi* and *Hysopus*, p. 52 below.

remote as might appear; in the section on stones, the names recorded by Albertus Magnus as *Peridonius*, *Gagatronica*, and *Hyaenia* were corrupted to *Feripendamus*, *Bagates*, and *Bena* respectively.

The most striking evidence of the popular, or unscholarly, nature of *The Book of Secrets* is not so much that the subject-matter is sensational, but that it is treated in a thoroughly unsophisticated manner. The magic recipes are greatly simplified, and involve none of the ritualistic complications normally associated with witchcraft, sorcery, alchemy, or medicinal magic. Sympathetic magic in its simplest form is the basis of many of the recipes; by what Frazer calls the 'Law of Similarity'[9] an object with certain attributes is thought to transfer these attributes to another object, simply by association with it. A particularly clear example of the logic of sympathetic magic can be seen in the *Kiranides*, a work with much in common with *The Book of Secrets*; of the nightingale it reports, 'If any will swallow down its Heart with Honey, while the bird is panting, and will carry about him the Heart and Tongue of the same Bird, he will be sweet in speech, and of shrill voice, and will be heard gladly.'[10] Similar logic can be seen in the magical qualities attributed to the wolf (p. 76), the stone *chalazia* (p. 44), and in the many recipes designed to effect the congregation of birds, animals, or fish (pp. 9, 52, and 55, for example). The theoretical introduction to the *Marvels of the World* (see pp. 74 ff.) explains in some detail the principles of sympathetic magic of this kind.

Although many of the recipes in *The Book of Secrets* have become so much simplified that it is impossible to trace their origin, some evidence of the original rituals has survived in a few cases. There is mention of an 'image' which will burn in water—a suggestion of the use of images in witchcraft (p. 106);

---

[9] Sir James G. Frazer, *The Golden Bough*, 3rd ed. (London, 1920), i. 54.

[10] *The Magic of Kirani King of Persia, and of Harpocration* (London, 1685), pp. 107–8.

the mention of 'a glass well spotted' (p. 98) refers to the use of sigils, or special designs, on articles used in the magic ritual; an incantation has apparently been omitted in a recipe con- cerned with the killing of serpents (p. 107); the association of herbs with particular astrological qualities may be an applica- tion of the 'doctrine of signatures', in which a plant's physical resemblance to an object—the moon, or an ear, for example— was thought to indicate a particular affinity for that object; and there are a number of recipes which may be garbled alchemical cryptograms, particularly that which refers to the salamander (pp. 53–4). However, even the recipes in which a magic ritual has survived are so vaguely recorded that it would have been impossible for a reader to put them into practice. One can only suppose that not even when the book was first compiled was it intended to be taken seriously as a handbook of magic; the author is interested in marvelling at those things that are written, rather than in putting them to the test.

And yet throughout *The Book of Secrets* there is emphasis on the importance of proof. There are the frequent assertions that 'this was proved in our time', a statement otherwise as un- necessary as untrue. There is the frequent use, in the Latin text, of the verb *experimentari* as well as *experiri*, 'experiment' rather than mere 'experience', and there is the introduction to the *Marvels of the World* which argues that natural properties should be discovered by experience and experiment rather than postulated theoretically, and that they should be proved by the evidence of the senses rather than by reason. Paradoxically, the argument for experiment is used to convince the reader that the manifestly untested recipes are workable, or at least to give the reader that edge of satisfaction in his reading by allowing him to believe that it just might be true. *The Book of Secrets* is an example of the medieval acceptance of authority in its most credulous form, coupled with the beginning of a questioning attitude; the writer did feel he had to claim that the recipes had been proved recently, even if they had not.

2. *The Book of Secrets* and the Elizabethans

If *The Book of Secrets* was unlikely to have been taken altogether seriously when it was written, by the time (*c.* 1550) it was translated into English it is even less likely that its readers would have believed literally everything it contained. The preface to the first English edition recommends that the book should be treated as light reading, like the 'Book of Fortune', a reference to the many almanacs and books of popular astrology available to the Elizabethan reader (see p. 2 below). However, by the edition of 1617 the printer felt it necessary to go further. He begins by making the same point as the earlier editions: 'Wherefore, use this Book for thy recreation (as thou art wont to use the book of Fortune) for assuredly there is nothing herein promised but to further thy delight', suggesting, incidentally, that the almanacs were not taken altogether seriously. But the preface continues with an almost apologetic scepticism: 'I refer thee to the trial of some of his secrets, which as thou shalt find true in part or all, I leave to thine own report or commendation' (sig. A. ii^v). An earlier comment on one recipe in *The Book of Secrets* assumes in the same way that readers will want to put the 'secret' to the test. Thomas Lupton, in his collection *A Thousand Notable Things of Sundry Sorts* (*c.* 1579), quotes *The Book of Secrets* frequently; he records (Book VII, No. 39) one of the recipes for holding fire in the hand unhurt (see p. 89 below), and then adds laconically, 'Praise it as it proves.'

A Thousand Notable Things is, as its name suggests, a contemporary Elizabethan anthology of 'marvels' very similar to *The Book of Secrets*. In 'The Preface of the Author to the Reader' Lupton attempts at some length to provide justification for such works; his argument is very simply that they provide recreation through variety:

... in my judgement, through the strangeness and variety of matter it will be more desirously and delightfully read, knowing that we are made of such a mould that delicate Daintiness delights us much, but we loathe to be fed too long with one food; and that long wandering in strange, pleasant and contrary places, will less weary us, than short travel in often trodden ground.

The readers of *A Thousand Notable Things* and *The Book of Secrets* were to be diverted and entertained by the exotic and varied subject-matter; the fact that both Lupton and the printer of the 1617 edition of *The Book of Secrets* assumed that the readers might go farther and actually try the 'secrets' for themselves suggests that they also possessed some curiosity and scepticism—qualities which would eventually lead to the death of a literature so firmly grounded on the improbable.

Further indication of the kind of audience which was attracted to *The Book of Secrets* may be gathered from what we can learn of the translator. True to the tradition of popular literature, he was no scholar; certainly the Latin text he was working from was corrupt (for examples look at the notes to *schistos*, pp. 39–40, *virites*, p. 42, and *chelonites*, p. 34, where we can compare with Albertus Magnus's original) but nevertheless he frequently mistranslated or misunderstood the Latin. The best example of this is in the introduction to the *Marvels of the World*, where we must assume that he did not understand the argument, since the distinction between the evidence of the senses and conclusions arrived at by reason is never made clear, nor are the distinctions between 'experience', 'experiment', and 'proof' in the Latin text retained in the English. The translator also relied heavily on the Latin–English dictionary compiled by Sir Thomas Elyot and Thomas Cooper (see below, p. xliv). The most disarming moment in the whole book is the occasion when a stone is described as being found in Britain, and the translator adds a digression: 'the most noble Isle of the world, wherein is contained both countries, England and Scotland' (p. 45); but even this is taken from Elyot's dictionary verbatim. That the translator had no intellectual pretensions is borne out also by the style of the English. The pedestrian nature of the style is inherited, in part, from the Latin, which tends to be made up of a series of simple sentences and clauses joined by conjunctions. But the style cannot be blamed altogether on the original; already by the second edition of the work extensive changes were made to vary the monotonous phrases of the first edition (see, for some examples, p. xlv below), and this process of revision continued with the later editions.

The most interesting way in which the translator's personality emerges is in his tendency to censor the original. He carefully omitted references to necromancy in the introduction to the *Marvels of the World*, reducing the length of the discussion by about half; and he omitted a large number of recipes, at least some because he must have disapproved of them, since most have to do with aphrodisiacs on the one hand, and contracep-tives—not one of which he translated—on the other. In the passage on the stone *magnes*, the text, following Albertus Magnus closely, concludes, in our translation: 'Moreover, if this stone be put brayed and scattered upon coals, in four corners of the house, they that be sleeping shall flee the house, and leave all' (see p. 26). In the Latin text, however, the final sentence continues, revealing the whole point of the operation, 'and then the thieves steal whatever they want.'

If the translator of *The Book of Secrets* judged his audience correctly, the book would have appealed to those who, while seeking recreation in the delights of the exotic, were nevertheless somewhat moralistic, at the same time content that their reading had little scholarly value. It is probable therefore that most buyers of *The Book of Secrets* came from the lowest class of the literate, and that the book was one of many exploiting the new markets opened up by the introduction of the printing press seventy-five years earlier. The nature of this audience is discussed at length in Louis B. Wright's *Middle-class Culture in Eliza-bethan England* (Cornell University Press, 1935), where *The Book of Secrets* is mentioned (p. 562) in a chapter that deals more fully with collections of 'secrets' of a rather more scholarly nature. Wright concludes that these books 'are typical of an enormous literature supplying middle-class readers with in-formation similar to that purveyed by modern magazines that traffic in science and pseudo-science' (p. 571). In our present age of wider literacy the equivalent level of taste would be well above the semi-literate; close, perhaps, to the kind of audience now enjoyed by the *Reader's Digest*. The middle-class Citizen's Wife in Beaumont and Fletcher's *The Knight of the Burning Pestle* is an entertaining target for satire because her combina-tion of naïvety and pretension to knowledge and status is the more absurd in one who should know better. She recommends homely semi-magic recipes and cures of a kind not very different from some of those in *The Book of Secrets*:

Faith and those chilblains are a foul trouble; Mistress *Merriethought*, when your youth comes home, let him rub all the soles of his feet, and the heels, with a mouse skin, or if none of your people can catch a mouse, when he goes to bed, let him roll his feet in the warm embers, and I warrant you he shall be well, and you may make him put his fingers between his toes and smell to them, it's very sovereign for his head if he be costive.[11]

Though the dramatists did not always treat the literature of secrets so ironically; Rowley and Middleton, in *The Changeling*, dramatize a magical test of virginity (more delicate than that given on p. 45 below) in such a way that it is obvious that the audience is at least expected to suspend disbelief (IV. i and IV. ii).

It would be wrong, therefore, to assume that *The Book of Secrets* interested only the lowest stratum of literate Elizabethan society; the belief of the Elizabethans in magic and superstition was widespread, and interest was almost universal. Stimulated by the representation of ghosts, magicians, and witches on the stage, much has been written about Elizabethan attitudes to magic, demonology, and witchcraft; we remember that witch-hunting reached its peak in England in the seventeenth century under James I, the author of a book on *Daemonologie* (1597), and we remember the seriousness with which Queen Elizabeth took her Court Astrologer, Dr. John Dee.[12]

[11] III. iii. 188–95, *Dramatic Works*, ed. Fredson Bowers (Cambridge, 1966).
[12] See Don Cameron Allen's informative work, *The Star-crossed Renaissance*

Madelaine Doran, in an article 'On Elizabethan "Credulity"' (*Journal of the History of Ideas*, i (1940), 151–76), has suggested that there were different 'levels' at which the Elizabethans would have reacted to the marvellous, from complete acceptance to 'complete rejection of the potential actuality of the phenomenon in question, yet a willingness for reasons of convention or of symbolism to entertain the fiction imaginatively'. The existence of *The Book of Secrets* might lead us to speak of a further level: complete rejection, yet a willingness to be entertained by the strange and improbable.[13]

   That an interest in the literature of secrets must have extended to those of appreciably more than minimal intellectual respectability can be shown by the casual jottings of two wellknown Elizabethans: Philip Henslowe, the financier who controlled the acting company which was the chief rival of Shakespeare's company, and Gabriel Harvey, a graduate of Oxford, and a strenuous pamphleteer. In Henslowe's *Diary*, in between the records of contracts with his actors and lists of money received for the presentation of the plays, there appear a number of miscellaneous items; a card trick, an astrological numbertrick, and a collection of recipes not so far removed from *The Book of Secrets*. For example:

> A medicine for deafness in the
> ears which hath been proved

Take ants' eggs and stamp [pound] them and strain them through a cloth, then take swine's grease [probably a misreading of the plant name

(Durham, N.C., 1941); Katharine M. Briggs, *Pale Hecate's Team* (London, 1962); Wallace Notestein, *A History of Witchcraft in England from 1558 to 1718* (New York, 1965); Robert R. Reed Jr., *The Occult on the Tudor and Stuart Stage* (Boston, Mass., 1965); and Robert H. West, *The Invisible World* (Athens, Ga., 1939). The most informative Elizabethan account is Reginald Scot's *The Discoverie of Witchcraft* (1579, reprinted Centaur Press, 1964).

[13] Passages from *The Book of Secrets* appear in a surprisingly wide variety of contemporary works, illustrating further the breadth of its appeal. Thomas Lupton (see p. xviii), Michael Scott (p. 60), Thomas Moulton (p. 63), Sir Hugh Platt (p. 89), William Baldwin (p. 98), and Thomas Hill (p. 100) all quote *The Book of Secrets*, some sceptically, some ironically, and some seriously.

'swine's cress'] or knotgrass, stamp the same and take the juice and mix [it] with the other straining of the eggs and put into the ear certain drops. It will help [also] old deafness, if God permit.[14]

'Ants' eggs' are credited with a different property on p. 88 below. In the same book, though not in Henslowe's hand, there is some real magic: 'Write these words in virgin parchment with the blood of a bat, upon Tuesday morning betwixt five or six in the morning or at night: "halia J.K. turbutzi", and tie it about thy left arm, and ask what ye will have.'[15] For recipes using bat's blood and incantations, see p. 107 below. Another remedy calls, in part, for 'The urine of a boy being an innocent'.

Gabriel Harvey's interest was a little more sophisticated. In a book called *A Most Excellent and Perfect Homish Apothecarye* . . ., translated from the German of H. von Braunschweig by John Hollybush, and published at Cologne in 1561, Harvey made a large number of manuscript notes. The book itself consists of medical recipes of the usual kind, more explicit than those in *The Book of Secrets*, and referring to more genuine sources, but to a modern eye unlikely to be any more effective: 'Macer writeth that the roots of peony be very good for the falling sickness [epilepsy] if they be hanged about the neck' (B. ii). Of greatest interest, however, are two blank pages which Harvey has filled with remedies he has himself collected:

A special good medicine & precious, against the cough, phthisic, wheezing in the breast; to comfort all spiritual parts of a man, the head, the heart, stomach, liver, & lights.

Take fleur-de-lis, smallage, lovage, radish, liquorice, saxifrage, half an handful of either of them: of stammarrh & fennel of each a full handful. Stamp them well together, & after steep them 24 hours in a quart of good vinegar: & put to them a pottle of fair running water: & seethe them till half be consumed. And then strain it through a linen cloth: & put thereto a pint of stone honey; & then purify all again on the fire; & stir

[14] *Henslowe's Diary*, ed. R. A. Foakes and R. T. Rickert (Cambridge, 1961), p. 40. Swine's cress (*Coronopus squamatus*) and knotgrass (*Polygonum aviculare*) are superficially similar creeping plants which are weeds of cultivated ground.
[15] Ibid.

it all together. Drink 2 spoonfuls thereof morning, & evening: & you shall not fail to find great ease.[16]

The difference between this and the remedies collected by Henslowe, or represented in *The Book of Secrets*, is considerable. The directions given are accurate, informative, and obviously meant to be used; the mixture itself, while unlikely to prove quite the cure-all Harvey suggests, is certainly not harmful, and might in truth give some ease. However, the page of manuscript notes which follows has this entry:

To know every complexion according to the signs & planets whereof they come, by judgement of sores . . .

If the sore be red, & hard, it is engendered of red choler, & is hot and dry.

His signs are Aries, Leo, & Sagittarius: his planets ☉ [the sun], & ♂ [Mars]. While the moon is in any of these signs, do no medicine, or plaster to it . . .

Again there is greater sophistication, as Harvey is following the Galenic doctrine of the four humours (sanguine, choleric, melancholic, and phlegmatic) corresponding to the four elements (air, fire, earth, and water, respectively), themselves defined by combinations of the four basic qualities, hot, cold, dry, and moist. But in extending this framework to include astrology, and in fact to be guided by it, Harvey joins many of his contemporaries in applying principles derived theoretically in one discipline to another (to us quite unrelated) area. The

---

[16] From blank pages facing the title-page of *A . . . Homish Apothecarye* now in the British Museum. These notes are not collected in G. C. Moore-Smith's *Gabriel Harvey's Marginalia* (Stratford-upon-Avon, 1913), though others of a similar nature are recorded—see p. 129, for example. Fleur-de-lis (*Lilium candidum*), smallage (*Apium graveolens*), lovage (*Ligusticum scoticum*), radish (*Raphanus sativus*), liquorice (*Glycyrrhiza glabra*), saxifrage (*Saxifraga granulata*), stammarrh (possibly gum dammar, *Agathis dammara*), fennel (*Foeniculum vulgare*) are all strongly flavoured and aromatic, and thus suitable for a linctus, except *Lilium* (which has obvious religio-magic properties) and *Saxifraga*, which was regarded as a remedy for 'stone', by the doctrine of signatures, because of the small granular swellings on the roots.

Elizabethans did not compartmentalize their knowledge; as the philosophical concept of the four basic qualities and elements formed the basis of all pursuits in natural science—in alchemy, in the herbals and bestiaries, in medical science, astrology, and psychology—so the various areas of human knowledge were felt to be parts of a harmonious whole rather than separate, possibly conflicting disciplines. Each study in its microcosm reflected the macrocosm of an ordered universe; even magic and witchcraft could be made to fit the over-all pattern. The debate for and against astrology is too complex a question to be considered here; what we can learn from Harvey's interest, and from the interest of his brother Richard,[17] is that the intellectual boundaries of superstition were set in a very different way from ours. Gabriel Harvey was being neither superstitious nor unorthodox when he fitted astrology into the pattern of medicine; and when a mind as informed and sceptical as his makes this transition so easily, we can begin to understand why simplified astrology and simplified medicine—the 'secrets'—were received so widely. Harvey, no less than the modern reader, would probably have considered *The Book of Secrets* a work of superstition, but his reasons for thinking so would have differed from ours.

The unity of the Elizabethan's universe was achieved by arranging facts to fit the over-all theory, by seeking resemblances rather than by testing differences. This is the deductive (as opposed to inductive) method of reasoning attacked by Bacon in his *Novum Organum* and *The Advancement of Learning*,[18] and described by the writer of the *Marvels of the World* as inadequate (see below, pp. 82 f.). The tendency to look to authority and theory for answers to specific problems, instead of looking to experience and experiment, was a habit of thought deeply ingrained in the minds of all but the most radical thinkers.

[17] See Allen, *The Star-crossed Renaissance*, pp. 121 f.

[18] See the *Novum Organum*, ed. Joseph Devey (New York, 1901); the *Selected Works*, ed. Sidney Warhaft (Toronto, London, 1965) contains relevant selections, and also includes *The Advancement of Learning*; see pp. 223–35 in particular.

There was one particularly interesting, though minor, pamphlet controversy between 1631 and 1637 which demonstrates very clearly this mental set.

In 1631 appeared *Hoplocrisma-spongus; or a Sponge to Wipe Away the Weapon-salve*, by William Foster, a parson, and graduate of Oxford; it was replied to a few months later by Dr. Robert Fludd, an eminent physician, Rosicrucian, and writer of a kind of medical mysticism which is the logical extension of the attitude we have already seen in Gabriel Harvey. Fludd's work was called *Doctor Fludds Answer unto M. Foster; or the Squeesing of Parson Fosters Sponge*. The controversy concerned an ointment, the 'weapon-salve', which was supposed to cure wounds by semi-miraculous means. The nature of the weapon-salve, and the way it worked, may be seen in a later contribution to the controversy, *The Weapon-salves Maladie: or, a Declaration of its Insufficiencie to Perform what is Attributed to it*, translated from the *Practice of Medicine* by 'the learned and judicious physician Daniel Sennertus, doctor and public Professor at Wittenberg'. Citing Johannes Baptista Porta and Paracelsus, the writer describes the weapon-salve thus:

> If the weapon which hath wounded anyone shall be brought, or a stick dipped in the same blood; the affected person shall be cured, although he be distant far away:

> Take *Moss* or *Scurf* (that groweth thick on a man's skull, left to the open air), and *Man's fat*, of each two ounces,
> *Mummy* and *Man's blood*, of each half an ounce,
> *Linseed Oil*, *Turpentine*, and *Bole Armeniac*, of each one ounce.

Let all these things be brayed [pounded] together in a mortar, and kept in a long and narrow pot. Dip the weapon into the unguent, and there let it lie: let the person hurt, in the morning cleanse his wound with his own water [urine]; and so bind it up, without anything else put to it, and the wounded person shall be cured without any pain.[19]

---

[19] See pp. 2-3. Porta's original appeared later in English as his *Natural Magic* (1658), which has been reprinted by Basic Books (New York, 1957);

The fascinating thing about the controversy between Foster and Fludd is that Foster attacks the weapon-salve not because it does not work, but because it is clearly (in his opinion) witch-craft, and the healing is therefore done by the agency of the Devil. The attack is made in the same philosophical framework as that which produced the weapon-salve itself, based as it is on deduction and the appeal to authority; it is no wonder, there-fore, that Dr. Fludd is able to defend the weapon-salve with as much, if not more, energy, since argument by analogy and the appeal to authority are highly adaptable methods for the making of a point. Foster tried to argue that the weapon-salve's working at a distance from the wound, not by contact with it, was an indication that it was unnatural:

Whatsoever worketh naturally, worketh by corporal or virtual contact; but this worketh by neither: *ergo* it worketh not naturally.

Thus Dr. Fludd quotes Master Foster ('virtual contact' refers to the natural powers, or 'virtues' of an object); Fludd then replies:

First, concerning that axiom in Philosophy, I know and can prove it by experience to be false. For the fire heateth *ad distans* ['at a distance']: the lightning out of the cloud blasteth *ad distans*. The baytree operateth against the power of thunder and lightning *ad distans* . . . the sun and fire do act in illuminating *ad distans*. The loadstone [magnet] doth operate upon the iron *ad distans*. The plague, dysentery, smallpox, infect *ad distans*, etc.[20]

And so it goes on; one feels that Doctor Fludd gets much the better of the battle. Sennertus, in *The Weapon-salves Maladie*, is on safer ground where his attack is on the more modern-

see pp. 288–9. Moss or lichen grows on bones exposed in moist situations, fragments of mummy were powdered or liquefied, and bole armeniac was a fine clay from Armenia. See also Sir Kenelm Digby's *A Late Discourse* . . . *Touching the Cure of Wounds by the Powder of Sympathy* (1658), and Allen G. Debus, *The English Paracelsians* (London, 1965).

[20] Both passages are taken from *Doctor Fludds Answer*, pp. 28–9.

sounding point that the weapon-salve is not the proven cause of the cure:

For many things may be conjoined with the effect, which are not the cause of it; so that, as it followeth not, 'While this man was walking it lightened, therefore his walking is the cause of the lightning', so it follows not, 'This wounded man is healed, and hath used the *weapon-salve*, therefore the *weapon-salve* is the cause of his healing' (p. 14).

From this it is only one step to the controlled experiment. The weapon-salve must have been well known as late as the Restoration, for it actually makes an appearance on stage in Dryden and Davenant's curious and extravagant fantasy based on *The Tempest*, *The Enchanted Island*, printed in 1670. Ferdinand duels with Hippolito, 'one that never saw Woman', and Hippolito is seriously injured. Ariel instructs Prospero to 'Anoint the Sword which pierc'd him with this Weapon-Salve, / And wrap it close from Air', and in a subsequent scene Miranda administers the potion, to the sword, with dramatic effect:

Hip. O my wound pains me.
Mir. I am come to ease you.

> [*She unwraps the Sword*

Hip. Alas! I feel the cold Air come to me,
My wound shoots worse than ever.

> [*She wipes and anoints the Sword*

Mir. Does it still grieve you?
Hip. Now methinks there's something laid just upon it.
Mir. Do you find no ease?
Hip. Yes, yes, upon the sudden all the pain
Is leaving me . . .[21]

To balance the extremism of Fludd, we should remember that at the same time as he was writing, attitudes of a thoroughly scientific nature were developing. There was Francis Bacon, for example, who may have had *The Book of Secrets* in mind when he wrote: 'In natural history we see there hath not been that

---

[21] *Shakespeare Adaptations*, ed. Montague Summers (London, 1922, reprinted Benjamin Blom, 1966), pp. 93, 96. See also the note to p. 95, on pp. 259–60.

choice and judgement used as ought to have been; as may appear in the writings of Plinius, Cardanus, Albertus, and divers of the Arabians, being fraught with much fabulous matter, a great part not only untried, but notoriously untrue.'[22] William Harvey published *De Motu Cordis*, establishing for the first time that the blood circulated through the body, instead of, as Aristotle and Galen had believed, moving back and forth separately in the arteries and veins. Earlier, William Gilbert, also a physician, published a work on the magnet, or loadstone (*De Magnete*), in 1600, in which he described the properties of the magnet as they could be discovered by experiment; his source of inspiration was the 'foundrymen, miners, and navigators with whom he had personal contacts'.[23] One such navigator, Robert Norman, discovered the dipping effect of the magnetic needle, and published his observations on it in *The Newe Attractive* (1581); his introduction 'To the Reader' states concisely the nature of the movement from authority to experience which was taking place:

Many and divers ancient authors, Philosophers and others, have written of the *Magnes* or *Loadstone*, as also of his substance, virtue, and operation, and thereupon setting down their opinions and judgements, have left the same as infallible truths for them that should succeed. And as I may not, nor mean not herein willingly to condemn the learned or ancient writers, that have with great diligence laboured to discover the secrets of Nature in sundry things . . . yet I mean, God willing, without derogating from them, or exalting myself, to set down a late experimented truth found in this Stone, contrary to the opinions of all them that have heretofore written thereof. Wherein I mean not to use barely tedious conjectures or imaginations, but briefly as I may to pass it over, founding my arguments only upon experience, reason, and demonstration, which are the grounds of Arts. (Sig. B. i.)

[22] *The Advancement of Learning*, ed. cit., p. 228.
[23] E. Zilsel, 'The Sociological Roots of Science', *American Journal of Sociology* (1941–2), reprinted in *Origins of the Scientific Revolution*, ed. Hugh Kearney (London, 1964), p. 95. For an admirable summary of scientific developments in England in the sixteenth century, see *The Development of Natural History in Tudor England*, by F. D. and J. F. M. Hoeniger (Folger Booklets on Tudor and Stuart Civilization, University Press of Virginia, 1969).

This last phrase we would read 'experience, reason, and demonstration (experiment), which are the basis of science'. Perhaps the most revealing thing about this passage, however, is the extent to which Norman felt obliged to apologize for daring to contradict authority.

Men like Bacon, William Harvey, Gilbert, and Norman were, however, the exceptions, for few of the Elizabethans were interested in experiment. It is not only the extent of the literature of secrets that makes us realize the fundamentally medieval cast of mind of the Elizabethan reader, it is the way that literature of a similar kind permeates a host of other subjects, popular and intellectual: the many books of medicine and astrology; the cookery books, which switch disconcertingly from appetizing recipes to horrifying remedies; the handbooks of husbandry, farming, gardening, even those on hawking and hunting. That people like Henslowe, Gabriel Harvey, Foster, and Fludd were interested in such secrets demonstrates that the fascination of the occult was not limited to the 'groundlings'; *The Book of Secrets* may indeed have been read mainly by the unsophisticated, but greater sophistication produced, for the most part, only a more complex treatment of the same kind of material. The Elizabethan age is usually thought of in the context of the Renaissance, as a time of re-birth, expansion, exploration, both of new countries and new ideas; but it is salutary to be reminded of the extent to which old ideas persisted, and to be reminded that the Elizabethans still retained much of the paradoxical combination of scepticism and credulity that we find in *The Book of Secrets* at the close of the thirteenth century.

3. The Background of Ideas and the Development of Natural Science

It is impossible to do justice to the history of natural science in a few pages; the discussion which follows is a summary of the most important developments in the areas of knowledge touched on in *The Book of Secrets*, with further reading suggested in the notes.

Two major figures, Hippocrates and Aristotle, may conveniently be taken as illustrating the beginning of natural science as we know it.[24] Hippocrates (b. 460 B.C.) was the leader of a school of medicine which was chiefly remarkable for its rejection of the idea of divine interference in the progress of disease and ill health, and its belief in the power of nature to perform cures with the aid only of appropriate diet, rather than medicine. Aristotle (384–322 B.C.), often thought of as primarily a philosopher, in fact carried out highly original work in the field of natural history. In his zoological studies his method was basically inductive, arguing from close observation of the animals he discusses to the establishment of general theories; his knowledge of the anatomy and structure of animals, especially those of the sea shore, was extensive and accurate, but he knew surprisingly little of their functions and behaviour. His information about even such a familiar animal as a mouse, for instance, was so scanty that he could write of it that it bore several hundred offspring at a single birth. He had a flair for recognizing essential similarities in the anatomical characteristics of animals, and produced the rudiments of a workable classification, the development of which much later, especially by Linnaeus in the eighteenth century, proved to be an essential for the development of modern biology. His division of animals into two major groups, those with and those without red blood systems, may be compared with the later division into vertebrates and invertebrates. Aristotle's

---

[24] Useful general histories of science are: Charles Singer, *From Magic to Science* (London, 1928) and *A Short History of Biology* (Oxford, 1931); *Ancient and Medieval Science*, ed. René Taton and trans. A. J. Pomerans (London, 1963); William T. Sedgwick and others, *A Short History of Science* (New York, 1939). Editions of Pliny, Aelian, Isidore, and Albertus Magnus are recorded in the list of 'Works Cited in the Notes to the Text', p. 113; the biological works of Aristotle and Theophrastus are published in the Loeb Classical Library, trans. A. L. Peck and Sir Arthur Hort, respectively; see also *The Greek Herbal of Dioscorides . . . Englished by John Goodyer A.D. 1655*, ed. Robert T. Gunther (New York, 1933).

pupil, Theophrastus (372–287 B.C.), continued the tradition
of observation, turning his attention to botany. His pioneering
work involved the description of more than 500 plant species,
together with their medicinal properties, and in addition he
made important observations on the anatomy and reproduction
of plants.

Later writers brought a different attitude to their work. A
tradition of the 'authority' gradually became established, and it
was thought preferable to compile uncritically the works of
earlier writers, rather than to contribute original observations.
This attitude can be seen developing in the field covered by
Theophrastus, the description of plants. Dioscorides (fl. *c.* A.D.
50), a military surgeon under Nero, compiled a work (*De
Materia Medica*), which remained the most important in its
field until the sixteenth century. Although he was both
methodical and accurate in his descriptions of plants, he was
not as original as Theophrastus. A contemporary of Dioscorides, Pliny the Elder (A.D. 23–79), illustrates more clearly the
change in attitude. His *Natural History* is an enormous and
informative compilation, but there is little evidence of personal
observation, and only in the more extreme cases does he show
any scepticism of the material he is reporting (see notes on pp.
35 and 52 for examples of his scornful attitude to the 'Magi').
For the most part Pliny passes on truth and fable with equal
seriousness. Two later encyclopedists, Aelian (A.D. 170–235)
and Isidore of Seville (A.D. 602–36), continue further the process
of uncritical reporting; since the texts from which these writers
worked were often corrupt, confusion was added to fable, and
the amount of real knowledge declined considerably.

It was not until the thirteenth century that a major writer
once again combined erudition with sufficient curiosity to lead
to accurate observation. Albertus Magnus (1206–79) has
already been discussed above as an example of a writer who
was typically medieval in his acceptance of authority—his
entire written output was intended as a commentary on
Aristotle—but who also was moved to compare the written

word to the real world, and to modify his beliefs in accordance with personal observation. Like Pliny and Isidore, Albertus Magnus also wrote at length on animals and minerals.

One other figure amongst the early natural scientists who should be mentioned here for the originality of his work is Galen (c. A.D. 129–200). Like the Hippocratic writers, Galen emphasized the value of diet and exercise in promoting health, though he also wrote at length on medicines. His knowledge of anatomy was very extensive, and undoubtedly based on personal observations, although he had an unfortunate tendency to assume that the structures he found in his dissections of, say, sheep, would also be found in other animals, and in particular, man. His work was unchallenged until 1543, when Vesalius in his *De Humani Corporis Fabrica* pointed out some of Galen's errors, at the same time, however, insisting on the correctness of the majority of his assertions.

The work of these writers, whether original or derived from authority, was a far cry from the popular literature of which *The Book of Secrets* is representative. The relationship between the scholarly and popular traditions can most conveniently be discussed in terms of the various sections of *The Book of Secrets*: herbs, stones, beasts, stars, and marvels.

(a) *The Herbals*. During the middle ages there were a large number of compilations, usually illustrated with woodcuts, which set forth the descriptions and the properties, real or supposed, of plants.[25] Their material was for the most part derived from Pliny and Dioscorides, though later authorities were often cited. There were a number of works, printed in Latin or German, and illustrated by woodcuts, which appeared soon after 1480: the *Herbarium* of Apuleius Platonicus

---

[25] See Agnes Arber, *Herbals, their Origin and Evolution* (Cambridge, 1938), from which much of the information in this section came; Sanford V. Larkey, ed., *An Herbal, 1525* (New York, 1941); Charles E. Raven, *English Naturalists from Neckham to Ray* (Cambridge, 1947); and Eleanor Rodhe, *The Old English Herbals* (London, 1922). Turner's short works on plants were reprinted by the Ray Society, ed. James Britten and others (London, 1965).

(*c.* 1481), a Latin *Herbarius* (1484), and a German *Herbarius* (1485) from which was derived the greater part of the section of the *Hortus Sanitatis* (1491) which deals with plants. In England two herbals of a similar kind were published: Richard Bancke's *Herball* (1525), later attributed by the printer, Robert Wyer, to Macer, without justification (see note, p. 16), and an anonymous work, *The Grete Herball* (1526). All of these herbals deal principally with the medical properties of the plants described, and depend far more on authority than on any original observation. Nevertheless, it was intended that the reader would be enabled to collect the herbs for himself for medicinal purposes, and the presence of illustrations, however crude initially, indicates that there was a growing interest in the plants themselves. Agnes Arber argues convincingly that it was the artist Hans Weiditz, illustrating a herbal by Otto Brunfels (1530), who started the movement back to the direct observation of nature, by his beautiful and accurate pictures of the plants. The Germans Hieronymus Bock and Leonhart Fuchs were the first to transfer the interest in real (as opposed to literary) plants to the text of the herbal.

In England the pioneer was William Turner (*c.* 1510–68). He published two small works of great importance to English botany, *Libellus de Re Herbaria Novus* (1538) and *The Names of Herbes in Greke, Latin, Englishe, Duche and Frenche* (1548), and followed these with his *Herball* in three parts, the first published in 1551, the second in 1562, and the third in 1568. Most of the illustrations are taken from the work of Leonhart Fuchs, but the text is full of vigour, originality, and a scorn for the accumulated superstitions of herbal literature. Another important work was the *Herball* (1597) of John Gerard (1545–1607). Gerard seems to have part-pirated, part-translated and somewhat rearranged the work of the great Belgian naturalist Rembert Dodoens; he himself contributed little to the work. The transition from the semi-popular, derivative early herbals to the scholarly and original work of Turner, Dodoens, and many others was completed in a remarkably short time; it was not much later that botany in the modern sense was established by figures like John Ray (c. 1627–1705).

One rather anomalous figure deserves mention: Nicholas Culpeper (1616–54), who published *A Physical Directory* in 1649, was an exponent of astrological botany, of a kind not notably superior to that recorded in *The Book of Secrets* in the group of seven herbs 'after the mind of Alexander' (p. 18). Though he was viciously attacked by the College of Surgeons in his own day, more on account of his temerity in translating the *Pharmacopoeia* into English for the first time than because of his astrological leanings, his works were popular, especially his posthumously published *English Physician and Complete Herbal*, which has been reprinted many times, one edition as recently as 1961.

(b) *The Lapidaries.* Many early writers on herbs also wrote on stones. Theophrastus, Dioscorides, Pliny, and Isidore included a good deal of material on minerals in their works, again largely treating them from the mythological and medical point of view. Further material of a popular nature was recorded by 'Damigeron', the author of a work *De Virtutibus Lapidum* ('On the Powers of Stones'). From obscure origins, the work appears in Latin from the sixth century onwards. Some manuscripts associate with it the name 'Evax', either as author or as translator; a later lapidary in Latin verse by Marbod (1035–1123) uses Damigeron extensively, and was also associated with Evax. Marbod's poem was translated into other languages, and seems to have been particularly popular in French and English manuscripts.[26] There were also a number of Christian lapidaries dealing with the list of precious stones in the breastplate worn by the high priest of the Jews (Exodus 28: 17–21)

[26] The key work followed here, and elsewhere, is the translation by Dorothy Wyckoff of Albertus Magnus's *Book of Minerals* (Oxford, 1967); see also Joan Evans, *Magical Jewels of the Middle Ages and the Renaissance, Particularly in England* (Oxford, 1922); Joan Evans and Mary Sergeantson, *English Medieval Lapidaries*, E.E.T.S., Orig. Ser. No. 190 (London, 1933); Paul Studer and Joan Evans, *Anglo-Norman Lapidaries* (Paris, 1924); and Fernand D. de Mély, *Les Lapidaires de l'antiquité et du moyen âge*, 3 vols. (Paris, 1896–1902).

and the slightly different list given in Revelation 21: 19–21 as forming the foundations of the New Jerusalem. This topic has fascinated commentators down to the present day, including Robert Graves (*The White Goddess*, London, 1948).

Albertus Magnus, in the alphabetical lapidary in his *Mineralia* from which the section on stones in *The Book of Secrets* is derived, seems to have used all of these sources, though he may not have known them all directly. He probably used the work of similar encyclopedists, men like Arnold of Saxony and Thomas of Cantimpré, who had already codified —and corrupted—the originals. Aaron, cited as an authority by Albertus, and mentioned in *The Book of Secrets*, was the author of an 'unidentified but presumably . . . Jewish or Arabic work'.[27]

(*c*) *The Bestiaries*. The interest of writers in the Middle Ages in symbols rather than actualities is nowhere better illustrated than in the books of beasts.[28] From much the same sources as

[27] Wyckoff, p. 270. Evidence that medical practitioners retained an interest in ancient beliefs and methods until well after the Elizabethan period can be found in P. Pomet's *Histoire générale des drogues* (Paris, 1694), which was compiled largely from Dioscorides, Pliny, Galen, and *The Book of Secrets*. It was translated anonymously into English and published under the title *A Compleat History of Drugges* in 1712, with a dedication to 'Dr. Sloane' which says that the edition was prepared largely under his guidance. Sir Hans Sloane (1660–1753) had a long and conspicuously successful career in medicine. He was personal physician to Queen Anne, and President of the Royal College of Physicians (1719–35). His success rested to a great extent on his use of quinine for fevers and milk chocolate for consumption, rather than the traditional remedies of the ancients. He was also of course a great antiquary and collector, and his collections formed the basis of the British Museum. Several drawers from a medicine chest belonging to him are in the possession of the British Museum (Natural History). The specimens in them appear to have been collected to illustrate the *History of Drugges* rather than for actual day-to-day use in his profession, for most of them are listed in the manuscript catalogue to his museum collection. It seems that Pomet's pharmacopoeia was already going out of fashion by the time it was translated into English, although on the other hand as late as 1745 Sloane was recommending an ointment made of 'viper's grease' admixed with such ingredients as powdered haematite, tutty (zinc oxide), and pearl.

[28] See Samuel A. Ives, *An English Thirteenth Century Bestiary* (New York, 1942); Montague R. James, ed., *The Bestiary . . . and a Preliminary Study of the*

the early herbals, there appeared a compilation associated with
the name 'Physiologus', perhaps originally some time between
the second and fifth centuries A.D. This work was modified and
expanded until it contained accounts of over a hundred beasts
in its most popular period, the twelfth century. The bestiary
typically gives a short description of an animal, often accom-
panied by a stylized illustration, and points a Christian moral
on some point of the animal's behaviour. The best-known
example of this is the pelican, which was said to lacerate its
breast to feed its young, and was thus a symbol of maternal
piety. In Physiologus, the legend was that the bird could revive
its young by piercing its breast and allowing its blood to pour
over their dead bodies; the obvious parallel was drawn with
Christ, who 'ascended to the height of the cross, and, his side
having been pierced, there came from it blood and water for
our salvation and eternal life'[29] (see p. 56 below).

The bestiary of Physiologus was never, so far as we know,
printed in England; the first major book on animals published
showed the same change in intellectual interest that we have
already seen in the herbals of Turner and Dodoens. Conrad
Gesner (1516–65) in his *Historiae Animalium* assembled an
enormous amount of learning combined with a basically
sceptical approach and a great deal of original observation of
the more familiar animals. A shortened version of this work
was translated into English by Edward Topsell and first
published in 1607 as the *Historie of Fourefootid Beastes*.

(*d*) *Astrology.* From the earliest times the studies we now
know as astronomy and astrology were thought of as a single
discipline.[30] From ancient beginnings in Babylonia several

Latin Bestiary as Current in England (Oxford, 1928); Albert S. Cook, ed. and
trans., *Old English Physiologus* (New Haven, Conn., 1921); Percy Ansell
Robin, *Animal Lore in English Literature* (London, 1932); Edward Topsell,
*The History of Four-footed Beasts and Serpents . . . Whereunto is Now Added, The
Theatre of Insects* [by Thomas Moffet] (London, 1658), reprinted, ed. Willy
Ley, 3 vols. (New York, 1967); T. H. White, trans., *The Book of Beasts*
(London, 1954).   [29] T. H. White, p. 133.
   [30] See Allen, *The Star-crossed Renaissance*; Walter C. Curry, *Chaucer and the*

centuries B.C., astronomy–astrology had already become complex and elaborate by the beginning of the Christian era.
Because of the association of the stars with pagan gods, the
Christian church at first opposed astrology, for theological
rather than scientific reasons; St. Augustine in *The City of God*
presents one of the most famous of these attacks.[31] After
Augustine, however, Christian thought became less inimical
to astrology, and in the thirteenth century both Albertus
Magnus and Thomas Aquinas accepted the concept of the
stars' influence on men's actions. They justified this by seeing
the stars as the instruments of God, intermediaries between the
First Mover and man, influencing him without robbing him
of free will. Although opposition to astrology persisted, the
sanction of the church was enough to ensure that astrological
writings multiplied. During the Elizabethan period an
enormous number of almanacs and treatises on astrology were
printed, and we have already mentioned the prominence of
Doctors Dee and Fludd. There are a number of Elizabethan
treatises explaining the complexities of the interaction between
planets and signs of the zodiac for the uninitiated reader; in
1556 Robert Recorde published the *Castle of Knowledge*, two
years later Fabian Wither published *Briefe Introductions unto the
Arte of Chiromancy, Whereunto is Annexed as Well the Artificiall
as Naturall Astrologie*, in 1581 there appeared John Maplet's
Diall of Destiny, and so on. Even Bacon, in his *De Augmentis
Scientiarum*, suggested that astrology should rather be 'purified
than altogether rejected'.[32] Since the seventeenth century,
astrology, separated from astronomy, has become a latter-day
popular literature, retaining sufficient following to justify
columns in newspapers and almanacs in supermarkets.

Medieval Sciences (London, 1926); Mark Graubard, *Astrology and Alchemy: Two
Fossil Sciences* (New York, 1953); Louis MacNeice, *Astrology* (London, 1964);
and Theodore O. Wedel, *The Medieval Attitude Towards Astrology* (London,
1911).   [31] Everyman Library ed. (1945), pp. 143 ff. (V. i–vii).

[32] *Works*, ed. James Spedding and others (Cambridge, 1863), vii. 489. The
original Latin text can be found in ii. 272; Bacon's earlier version in *The
Advancement of Learning* is less specific (see Warhaft edn., p. 229).

The astrology of *The Book of Secrets* is not much different from the astrology of today's newspaper columns. Whereas today we simplify by considering the signs of the zodiac only, *The Book of Secrets* in the Latin version simplifies by considering the influence of the planets only. Originally the only sections dealing with astrology were the section on the seven herbs of the seven planets, and the section explaining the hours of the day governed by the planets, placed after the section on beasts. The summaries of the qualities attributed to each planet were added in the later Elizabethan editions, probably because it was felt that the original comment was too sketchy to be of real interest. We have not been able to trace the source of this section; it could have been taken from any one of a large number of more detailed works on astrology published before 1590.

(e) *The Literature of 'Secrets'.* The origin of the literature of secrets lies ultimately in pre-Christian rites and religions of southern Europe, Northern Africa, and the Near East. There are the shadowy figures of the Magi, the Persian priest-magicians of Babylon, and Hermes Trismegistus, the name of a god-figure which was associated with a large body of magical, mystical, and alchemical writings.[33] The origin and date of these magical and semi-medical works are obscure, and in any case they must derive from an oral tradition of far greater antiquity. The variety and extent of the influence of the oral tradition may be gauged by the fact that *The Book of Secrets*, written, possibly in Cologne, at the close of the thirteenth century, records a number of recipes obviously related to this

[33] See Émile Benveniste, *Les Mages dans l'ancienne Iran*, Études Iraniennes, No. 15 (Paris, 1938); Patrick Boylan, *Thoth the Hermes of Egypt* (Oxford, 1922); Eric J. Holmyard, *Alchemy* (Harmondsworth, Middx., 1957); John Maxson Stillman, *The Story of Alchemy and Early Chemistry* (New York, 1960); and Frances A. Yates, *Giordano Bruno and the Hermetic Tradition* (London, 1964). On magic, in addition to works cited above in the section on 'The Book of Secrets and the Elizabethans', see Maurice Bouisson, *Magic, its History and Principal Rites* (London, 1960), and Grillot de Givry, *Witchcraft, Magic and Alchemy*, trans. J. Courtenay Locke (London, 1931).

one, found in the *Kama Sutra of Vatsyayana*, a Hindu treatise written some time between 300 B.C. and A.D. 300:

If a lamp, trimmed with oil extracted from the shrawna and priyangu plants (its wick being made of cloth and the slough of the skins of snakes), is lighted, and long pieces of wood placed near it, those pieces of wood will resemble so many snakes.[34]

See pages 17–18 and 102 below for similar 'perfumings'. Another work, *The Book of Medicines*, written in the 'early centuries of the Christian era' by 'a follower of one of the most advanced Schools of Medicine that flourished in Alexandria in the second century before Christ',[35] contains one section, in marked contrast with the scholarly nature of the rest of the work, which records specifically popular remedies, many of which are similar to those in *The Book of Secrets*. One, 'to make beetles depart from a house' reads, 'Throw into [the house] fresh roses, and they will flee' (ii. 688; compare p. 90 below).

The preface to *The Book of Secrets* before the section on herbs mentions the book of *Kiranides*, 'a book of uncertain date and authorship, usually called the *Kiranides* of Kiranus [or Cyranus], King of Persia'.[36] The kind of magic it contains is in many places very similar to that of *The Book of Secrets*, particularly the sections on herbs and beasts, but the actual recipes are different, and it was clearly not a source for *The Book of Secrets*.[37] The *Kiranides* was published in England as late as 1685 as *The Magick of Kirani King of Persia, and of Harpocration*, in a text with a carefully prepared index of the diseases mentioned and their 'cures'. It is available in Latin with a parallel translation in French in a text edited by L. Delatte (Liège, 1942). Appended to the book originally, it seems, were the seven herbs 'after the mind of Alexander' also found in *The Book of Secrets*; this may be why the *Kiranides*

[34] Trans. Sir Richard F. Burton (reprinted New York, 1964), p. 251. Both plant names refer to millet, *Setaria italica*.

[35] Sir Ernest A. T. W. Budge, *Syrian Anatomy, Pathology and Therapeutics, or 'The Book of Medicines'* (London, 1913), i. v.

[36] Thorndike, *History*, ii. 229.

[37] Thorndike, 'Further Consideration of the *Experimenta* . . .'.

is cited as a source in the preface. The seven herbs are more often said to be the work of a Flaccus Africanus or Alexius Affricus, writers otherwise unknown.

The book of *Alchorath* cannot certainly be identified; the translator's preface to the 1685 edition of the *Kiranides* quotes the preface of *The Book of Secrets* as evidence that Albertus Magnus approved of the *Kiranides*, and goes on to identify 'Alchorat' with 'Arpocrationis', Harpocration, or possibly Hippocrates—but even it this were true, it would of course be another spurious attribution. Elsewhere in the text the book of *Alchorath* is associated with the Hermetic writings (p. 54), but in the section on stones the reference (p. 46) is added by the compiler of the present text, for it is not explicitly mentioned by Albertus Magnus, who refers more vaguely to '[books on] incantations and physical ligatures' (Wyckoff, p. 90). Other writers who have not been identified are 'Architas' and 'Tabariensis', and the two sources 'Archigenis' and 'the book of Cleopatra' are almost unknown, though Galen cites both writers as sources. Achigenes 'practised in Rome in the reign of Trajan [A.D. 98–117] and wrote many medical works';[38] from the evidence of recipes in the Latin text attributed to it, we can guess that 'the book of Cleopatra' (as its name suggests) was probably concerned with aphrodisiacs and devices to promote or hinder conception, some of which, again, remind us of the recipes in the *Kama Sutra*. Very few of these recipes were translated into English. 'Belbinus' may, Thorndike suggests, be the same as the 'Belenus' cited in another work attributed to Albertus Magnus (the *Speculum Astronomiae*), and his name is also associated with the seven herbs 'after the mind of Alexander', as 'Flaccus Africanus' is represented as being one of his followers.[39]

The 'son of Messias' was probably Mesüe Junior (Masawija al-Marindi, d. 1015), who is supposed to have popularized Arabic medicine in Latin translations, but seems to have been

[38] Budge, ii. clxiv.
[39] Thorndike, *History*, ii. 234, 735.

'a most unreliable writer'.[40] That the school of Arabic medicine influenced both scholarly and popular literature is undoubted. The greatest of the Arabic physicians was Rhazes (Abu Bekr Muhammed ibn Zakarija ar-Razi, c. 841–926), but the most influential was Avicenna (Abu 'Ali Husayn ibn-'Abdullah ibn Sina, 987–1037), whose *Canon*, a million words in length, was the 'final codification of all Graeco-Arabic medicine', and was used in European universities as a textbook until 1650.[41] It has also been suggested that Avicenna was the author of the famous poem by 'Omar Khayyam'.

There are three names of considerable fame cited in *The Book of Secrets*, Plato, Aristotle, and Galen, but all are references to popular works erroneously attributed to these writers. The names of 'Plato' and 'Galen' are taken from one of the major sources of the *Marvels of the World*, a compilation known as the *Liber Vaccae*.[42] In our texts it is called the *Libri Tegimenti* or *Regimenti*; *tegimenti* might mean 'of defences' (against disease etc.), but *Libri Regimenti*, 'the book of rules' or 'government', is more plausible. The *Liber Vaccae* is attributed, without justification of course, to both Plato and Galen, hence the appearance of the names in *The Book of Secrets*. The references to the pseudo-Aristotle, likewise mentioned in the *Liber Vaccae*, involve another popular work, the *Secreta Secretorum*, or a similar work in the same tradition; these dealt with much the same kind of magic as the *Marvels of the World*, specifically relating it to Aristotle and Alexander the Great, to whom Aristotle was tutor (see p. 85 below).[43]

One further source of *The Book of Secrets* not mentioned in the text is the *Book of Fires* by Marcus Grecus, from which the various magical suffumigations and actual explosives towards

---

[40] Donald Campbell, *Arabian Medicine and its Influence on the Middle Ages* (London, 1926), i. 76–7.

[41] Campbell, i. 79 ff.

[42] It is known by several other titles—see Thorndike, *History*, ii. 778 ff., from which the information about this work was taken.

[43] See George Cary, *The Medieval Alexander*, ed. D. J. A. Ross (Cambridge, 1956).

the end of the *Marvels of the World* are taken. Again, who Marcus Grecus was is uncertain; the book seems to have been written not long before *The Book of Secrets*.[44] Another work of some importance is the *Hortus Sanitatis*. From origins as obscure as *The Book of Secrets* it was compiled in the fifteenth century and published in several languages, including, in an abbreviated version, English.[45] It is divided into sections on beasts, fowls, fish, serpents, and stones, and in the Latin version[46] the names of the animals are given in several languages, as in *The Book of Secrets*, but bear no relation to the apparently fictitious names in our text. The descriptions of the animals are at times realistic and accurate, but the 'operations' or properties ascribed to them are as magic as the recipes in the *Kiranides* and *The Book of Secrets*, both of which are frequently cited as authorities.

4. The Text

The texts of *The Book of Secrets* are many, and their history complicated. The first Latin manuscripts recorded by Thorndike in the *History of Magic and Experimental Science* date from the end of the thirteenth century, and from that time manuscripts proliferate. The first printed edition (in Latin) in the British Museum is dated *c.* 1470, and editions appear well into the sixteenth century. *The Book of Secrets* was translated into various languages, as the preface to the copy text points out; an Italian edition appeared in 1515, a French edition in about 1520, and the German text from which we have taken the woodcuts for the present edition was printed in 1548—and this list is by no means exhaustive. Editions in French persisted until 1937.

There are nine printed English texts of *The Book of Secrets*:

44 See Thorndike, *History*, ii. 252, 785 ff.
45 There is a German version, the *Gart der Gesuntheit*, by Johann von Cube, and a related Latin work, the *Herbarius*. See also *An Early English Version of the Hortus Sanitatis*, ed. N. Hudson (London, 1954), which reprints the original of Antwerp, *c.* 1521
46 *Ortus Sanitatis* (Morgantia, 1491).

three undated editions printed by William Copland, one un-dated edition printed by William Seres, four editions printed by William Jaggard, dated respectively 1595, 1599, 1617, and 1626, and one by T. Coates dated 1637.

The three Copland editions are the first, and must have been printed before *The Book of Secrets* was entered in the *Stationers' Register* to J. Kynge, as 'a boke Called *ALBERTUS MAGNUS*', on 30 August 1560. One edition (the copy text) has the date MDXXV on the title page, but this is clearly impossible, since William Copland did not start printing until about 1548. There is, moreover, internal evidence which allows us to establish that the date of printing was after 1545. In 1538 Sir Thomas Elyot, better known for his book on education, *The Governor*, published a dictionary translating from Latin to English; this dictionary was reissued in 1545, 1548, 1556, etc., 'inriched' by Thomas Cooper. The translator of the Latin text of *The Book of Secrets* leaned heavily on this dictionary, using many of its definitions verbatim. The follow-ing quotations establish that the edition used was that of 1545 or later:

Elyot 1538: Britayne, whiche doth contein Englande, Scot-lande, and wales.

Elyot 1545: Britania, is the moste noble yle of the worlde, wherin be conteyned bothe cuntreys Englād and Scot-lande . . .

The Book of Secrets: Brytannia, the moste noble Yle of the worlde, wherin is conteyned both countreis, England and Scotland. (D.v)

Elyot 1538: (no entry).

Elyot 1545: Stellio, a beaste lyke a lysarde, hauing on his backe spottes lyke starres.

The Book of Secrets: Stellio . . . which is lyke a lisard, hauing on his backe spottes lyke sterres . . . (E.iii^v)

These two entries are enough to show that the edition of 1538 was not used. There are two slight suggestions that the edition of 1548, which was further changed, was not used either: Elyot 1548 translates *hernioso* as a man that is 'brusten' while Elyot 1545 has the spelling 'brosten' of *The Book of Secrets* (I.iii); neither edition has an entry under *scrofula*, but the entry in 1545 under *scrofa* reads 'a sow that has pigges', from which the translator probably guessed the erroneous 'swyne pockes' (B.v etc.), while, also under *scrofa*, the entry in 1548 goes on 'or a disease called stuma', and under *stuma* explains that it is the disease known as the 'king's evil'.

We are left with the period 1545–60 for the Copland editions. Further evidence of a more slender nature suggests the period *c.* 1548–50 for the copy text. Two books, also published by Copland, of which we may be fairly sure of the dates, share with the copy text ornamental letters. *The True Dyfferēs between ye Regall Power and the Ecclesiasticall Power*, by Edward Fox, and *The Garden of Wysedome*, by Richard Taverner, have the same ornamental 'S' as *The Book of Secrets* (A.iv); *The True Dyfferēs* is dated 1548, and *The Garden of Wysedome* is found, in contemporary binding, with a translation (also by Taverner) of selections from Erasmus dated 1550.

It is not difficult to establish the order of the three Copland editions, the copy text (C1) in the British Museum, the second edition (C2) in the Huntington Library, and the third edition (C3) in the University Library, Cambridge. The many variant readings fall into two groups: those in which C1 and C2 are the same, and those in which C2 and C3 are the same, thus establishing C2 as the intermediate edition. The nature of many of the changes made in C2 and followed by C3 indicates clearly that these were later, as they tend either to modernize C1, or to reduce the monotony of its style by introducing variations in expression when a formula is frequently repeated. A few examples will illustrate this:

C1 (C.vii) has 'anone', C2 and C3 'straght'.
C1 (H.iii^v) has 'And they sayde', C2 and C3 'They sayd also'.

C1 (H.iiii) has 'And thei said', C2 and C3 'They say further'.

C1 (I.iiii) has 'And they saye', C2 and C3 'Further they say'.

C1 (I.iiii) has 'And they saye', C2 and C3 'Moreouer'.

Examples of readings in common with C1 and C2, not shared by C3:

C1 (D.v^v) has 'wasshen', C2 has 'washen', and C3 'washed'.

C1 (E.vii^v) has 'a cockes combe', C2 'a Cockes combe', and C3 'the Cockes combe'.

C1 (F.iii) and C2 have '.i. houre', C3 'an houre'.

C1 (G.vii^v) and C2 have 'chaunce', C3 'chaunge'.

There are also a number of occasions when C2, followed by C3, incorrectly 'corrects' C1:

C1 (B.ii) has 'Macer floridus', C2 'master Floridus', C3 'Master Floridus'.

C1 (D.vii^v) has 'bittes' [bites], C2 and C3 'bitternes'.

C1 (E.i^v) has 'owsel', C2 and C3 'Owle'.

C1 (E.vii^v) has 'geuethe', C2 and C3 'getteth'.

C1 (I.iiii^v) has 'mule', C2 and C3 'Mole'.

The editions of Jaggard, which follow the copy text, are of no bibliographical importance, except to show that the Elizabethan printers freely altered the text, no doubt because the prose seemed pedestrian. The edition of William Seres (S), recorded as being published in about 1570, is more interesting. It follows the copy text *literatim*, but corrects a number of errors in it rather more intelligently than C2. In at least four cases one is tempted to believe that a Latin text has been consulted:

C1 (A.viii^v) has 'which', followed by C2 and C3, while S has 'Witches' (Latin *magi*).

C1 (B.ii) has 'tasten', mis-corrected by C2 and C3 as 'taken', while S has 'casten' (Latin *coniecta*).

C1 (F.iv^v) has 'polayse', mis-corrected by C2 and C3 as 'polesy', while S has 'palaise' (Latin *palatium*).

And, most impressively, one of the foreign names is recorded by the copy text, and followed by C2 and C3, as 'Assifena' (A.vii^v), but this is changed in S to 'Esifena', the version recorded by all the Latin texts I have examined. It seems possible that Seres was able to print from a corrected version of C1; other occasions when S corrects C1 are recorded in the collation.

The present text was arrived at by detailed collation of the three editions printed by Copland and the one printed by Seres. Constant reference was made to the Latin text, particu-larly when the English text was obscure, but no attempt was made to correct the English text unless the sense of the passage was considerably improved—the 'swyne pockes' was left as 'swine pox' rather than corrected to 'scrofula', and the mis-translation is recorded in the notes. On points of interest several Latin texts were consulted; the edition used in the collation (described by Thorndike as one of the most correct, although the Latin is often corrupt) was *Liber aggregationis seu liber secretorum Alberti Magni* . . . printed by 'Wilhelmum de Mechlinia', in London ('*Juxta pontem qui vulgariter dicitur* Flete brigge'), *c.* 1485. The woodcuts of herbs and planets were taken from a German edition of 1548, *Naturalia Alberti Magni* . . . printed by I. Cammerlander in 'Strassburg'; the frontis-piece appeared in a Latin edition, *Liber Secretorum Alberti Magni* (Venitiis, 1502), and the picture of Albertus and a disciple experimenting with the dung of various animals comes from a French edition, *Les Admirables Secrets d'Albert le Graud* (Lyons, 1758). In addition, the woodcuts of animals and stones come from the *Hortus Sanitatis* (Morgantia, 1491), and the table of the 'hours and days' of the planets is taken from Robert Fludd's *Utriusque Cosmi Historia* (Oppenheim, 1617–18). All these are reproduced by the kind permission of the British Museum.

The text of the section on the seven planets which appears for the first time in the copies printed by Jaggard was taken from the edition of 1599 and collated with that of 1617. The earliest text, 1595, we have been unable to trace; it is recorded by the *Short Title Catalogue* as being in the possession of Captain Jaggard at Stratford-on-Avon, but his library has been sold, and we could find no record of *The Book of Secrets* in the records of the auctions.

The only section of *The Book of Secrets* which has a traceable and definite source is the section on stones, which was taken from the lapidary of Albertus Magnus in his *Mineralia* (ii. 2). Reference was made to the Latin text in the *Opera Omnia*, ed. Augusti Borgnet (Paris, 1890–9), and a number of readings, where the text was particularly obscure, were adopted from the translation of the *Mineralia* by Dorothy Wyckoff (*Book of Minerals*, Oxford, 1967).

In the present edition, spelling has been modernized both in the text and in quotations from contemporary sources. Punctuation, following the lead of the later Elizabethan editions, has been freely emended where necessary for the sake of clarity. The copy text fairly consistently capitalizes names of herbs, stones, and beasts, and we have retained this practice.

The book of secrets of Albertus Magnus
of the virtues of herbs, stones and certain beasts

Also, a book of the same author,
of the marvellous things of
the world: and of
certain effects, caused
of certain beasts

Sith it is manifestly known, that this book of Albertus Magnus is in the Italian, Spanish, French, and Dutch tongues, it was thought if it were translated into the English tongue, it would be received with like goodwill and friendship, as it is in those parts. Wherefore use thou this book to mitigate and alacrate thy heavy and troublesome mind, as thou hast been wont to do with the book commonly called the Book of Fortune: for believe me, whatsoever is promised in either of them both, this or that, is alonely to this end.

The Book of Secrets was translated into all the languages mentioned; the last French popular edition was published in this century, the last English edition in 1637. The translator suggests that the book should be treated as light reading like that offered by the fortune-telling astrological almanacs. To 'alacrate' is to enliven. The ascription of The Book of Secrets to Albertus Magnus is certainly false, although the section on stones is taken from one of his works.

The First Book of the Virtues of Certain Herbs

Aristotle, the Prince of Philosophers, saith in many places that 1
every science is of the kind of good things. But not withstand-
ing, the operation sometimes is good, sometimes evil, as the
science is changed to a good or to an evil end, to which it
worketh. Of the which saying, two things be concluded: the
one, and the first, is that the science of Magic is not evil, for by
the knowledge of it, evil may be eschewed, and good followed.
The second thing is also concluded, forasmuch as the effect is
praised for the end; and also the end of science is dispraised,
when it is not ordained to good, or to virtue. It followeth then,
that every science or operation is sometimes good, sometimes
evil. Therefore, the science of Magic is a good knowledge (as
it is presupposed) and is somewhat evil in beholding of causes
and natural things, as I have considered, and perceived in
ancient authors; yea, and I myself, Albert, have found the
truth in many things, and I suppose the truth to be in some part
of the book of *Kiranides*, and of the book of *Alchorath*.

First therefore I will declare of certain herbs, secondly, of 2
certain stones, and thirdly, of certain beasts, and the virtues
of them.

Heliotropium	Marigold
Urtica	Nettle
Virga pastoris	Wild Teasel

§ 1. Although knowledge ('science') may be considered basically good, it can
be perverted in its application ('operation') and be turned to evil ends; and
although there is potential danger in turning attention too closely to material
things, the truth can be found in magic as well as in more accepted studies.
The *Kiranides* is a work similar to *The Book of Secrets*, but not, apparently, used
as a source, and 'the book of *Alchorath*' may be a reference to Hippocrates (see
Introduction, p. xli).

Chelidonium	Celandine
Pervinca	Periwinkle
Nepeta	Calamint or Pennyroyal
Lingua canis	Hound's-tongue
Jusquiamus	Henbane
Lilium	Lily
Viscum querci	Mistletoe
Centaurea	Centaury
Salvia	Sage
Verbena	Vervain
Melissophyllum	Smallage
Rosa	Rose
Serpentina	Snake's-grass

3   The first herb is called with the men of Chaldea, *Elios*, with the Greeks, *Matuchiol*, with the Latins, *Heliotropium*, with Englishmen, Marigold, whose interpretation is of *helios*, that is the Sun, and *tropos*, that is alteration, or change, because it is turned according to the Sun. The virtue of this herb is marvellous: for if it be gathered, the Sun being in the sign *Leo*, in August, and be wrapped in the leaf of a Laurel, or Bay tree, and a Wolf's tooth be added thereto, no man shall be able to have a word to speak against the bearer thereof, but words of peace. And if any thing be stolen, if the bearer of the things before named lay them under his head in the night, he shall see the thief, and all his conditions. And moreover, if the aforesaid

§ 3. The supposed Aramaic and Greek names of these plants seem to be entirely fictitious (see Introduction, p. xv). *Heliotropium europaeum* was held by herbalists to be under the dominion of the sun; *Leo* is the sign of the zodiac associated with the sun. Turner (1548) says: 'They are foully deceived and shamefully deceive others which hold in their writings that our marigold is the *Heliotropium* of Dioscorides.' The marigold is *Calendula officinalis*, said by Culpeper (1669) to be also under the dominion of the sun. The bay tree is *Laurus nobilis*, a culinary rather than a medicinal herb. Perhaps *Prunus laurocera-sus*, the cherry laurel, whose leaves yield prussic acid on bruising, is meant here, and 'wolf's tooth' might refer to *Aconitum napellus*, a poisonous herb sometimes called 'wolfsbane', as both these plants were associated with the witch cult in medieval times. Sympathetic magic associated with the wolf is discussed on p. 76.

herb be put in any church where women be which have broken matrimony on their part, they shall never be able to go forth of the church, except it be put away. And this last point hath been proved, and is very true.

The second herb is called of the men of Chaldea *Roybra*, of 4

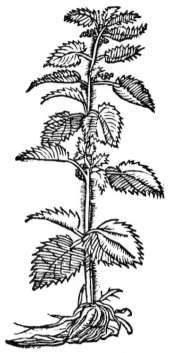

FIG. 1. *Urtica*, nettle.
From *Naturalia Alberti Magni* (1548)

§ 4. *Urtica dioica* is the common stinging nettle, but probably *U. pilulifera*, the so-called Roman nettle, a vigorous annual plant formerly widely cultivated in herb gardens, is intended here. *Achillea millefolium*, most commonly called yarrow, is still officinal in Central Europe as a tonic and stimulant. 'Nosebleed' is a local name in several parts of England, paralleled by the French *saigne-nez*; the three English names are taken from Elyot's Latin dictionary (1545). The magic of the houseleek, *Sempervivum tectorum*, is correlated with its manner of growth on roofs without any soil, and its evergreen habit. There is no reason to believe that any of these plants is attractive to fish, and why fish should come *ad piscellum* ('to the little fish') is obscure, though it may be a reference to the

the Greeks *Olieribus*, of the Latins or Frenchmen *Urtica*, of Englishmen a Nettle. He that holdeth this herb in his hand, with an herb called Milfoil, or Yarrow, or Nosebleed, is sure from all fear and fantasy, or vision. And if it be put with the juice of Houseleek, and the bearer's hand be anointed with it, and the residue be put in water; if he enter in the water where fishes be, they will gather together to his hands, and also *ad piscellum*. And if his hand be drawn forth, they will leap again to their own places, where they were before.

5   The third herb is named of the Chaldees *Lorumboror*, of the Greeks *Allamor*, of the Latins *Virga pastoris*, of Englishmen Wild Teasel. Take this herb, and temper it with the juice of Mandrake, and give it to a Bitch, or to another beast, and it shall be great with a young one in the own kind, and shall bring forth the birth in the own kind; of the which young one, if the gum tooth be taken and dipped in meat or drink, every one that shall drink thereof shall begin anon battle. And when thou would put it away give to him the juice of Valerian and peace shall be anon among them, as before.

6   The fourth herb is named *Aquilaris*, of Chaldees, because it springeth in the time in which the Eagles build their nests. It is named of Greeks *Valis*, of Latins *Chelidonium*, and of

phallus. Recipes for bringing about the miraculous assembly of various other animals are given later, see pp. 9, 13, and 55, for examples.

§ 5. The heads (teasels) of *Dipsacus fullonum*, the plant called here *virga pastoris* ('shepherd's rod'), are used for raising the nap on some kinds of woollen cloth. *Mandragora officinalis* (mandrake) was valued for its bizarrely branching rootstocks, which frequently resemble manikins, and were thought to scream when taken from the ground. Together with many other properties, mandrake was thought to increase fertility, and to be an aphrodisiac; taken with the hint in the Latin name for teasel (*virga*, literally 'a twig', acquired the meaning in late Latin of 'phallus'), this may explain the belief in the potency of the mixture. 'In the own kind' means 'in the same species'. Valerian (*Valeriana officinalis*) was said by Culpeper (1669) to be used as a mild narcotic.

§ 6. *Chelidonium majus* is the celandine or swallow-wort; Pliny (xxv. 50. 90) says it 'blossoms when the swallow arrives and withers when it departs'. The statement here that a man possessing this herb 'shall overcome . . . all matters in suit' is similar to the claim made later for the stone *chelidonius* (see p. 38) that it 'bringeth the business begun to an end'.

Englishmen Celandine. This herb springeth in the time in which the Swallows, and also the Eagles, make their nests. If any man shall have this herb, with the heart of a Mole, he shall overcome all his enemies, and all matters in suit, and shall put away all debate. And if the before named herb be put upon

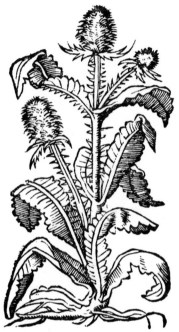

FIG. 2. *Virga pastoris*, wild teasel.
From *Naturalia Alberti Magni* (1548)

the head of a sick man, if he should die, he shall sing anon with a loud voice, if not, he shall weep.

The fifth herb is named of the Chaldees *Iterisi*, of the Greeks 7

§ 7. Culpeper mentions two kinds of periwinkle; he is referring to the two most commonly cultivated species, *Vinca minor* and *V. major*. They are, he says, owned by Venus, and 'the leaves eaten by man and wife together cause love between them'; like the houseleek (see note, p. 5), they are evergreen. In the north of England houseleek is sometimes called 'bullock's eye'; the 'beast called the Bugle' is a wild ox. The statement in the last sentence may have been suggested by the bright blue colour of the flowers of periwinkle.

Vorax, of the Latins *Proventalis*, or *Pervinca*, of Englishmen Periwinkle. When it is beaten unto powder with worms of the earth wrapped about it, and with an herb called *Semperviva*, in English Houseleek, it induceth love between man and wife, if it be used in their meats. And if it shall be put to the mouth

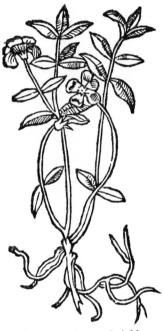

FIG. 3. *Pervinca*, periwinkle.
From *Naturalia Alberti Magni* (1548)

of the beast, called the Bugle, he shall break anon in the middle. And this was proved of late time. If the said confection be put in the fire, it shall be turned anon unto blue colour.

8   The sixth herb is named of the Chaldees *Bieith*, of the Greeks

§ 8. *Nepeta cataria*, catmint, and *Mentha pulegium*, pennyroyal, are both, according to Culpeper, 'under the dominion of Venus'. Turner regards them as kinds of calamint, but Culpeper says *Calamintha* is 'under the dominion of Mercury'. Probably *Mentha pulegium*, which was regarded virtually as a panacea until long after the end of the Middle Ages and was officinal in the *British Pharmacopoeia* as late as 1867, is the plant intended. The stone found in the nest of the lapwing is

Retus, of the Latins *Nepeta*, of Englishmen Calamint, otherwise Pennyroyal. Take this herb and mix it with the stone found in the nest of the bird called a Lapwing, or Black Plover, and rub the belly of any beast, and it shall be with birth, and it shall have a young one, very black in the own kind. And if it be put to their nostrils, they shall fall to the ground anon as dead, but a little space after they shall be healed. Also if the aforesaid confection be put in a vessel of Bees, the Bees will never flee away, but they shall gather together there. And if the Bees be drowned and like as they were dead, if they be put in the afore-said confection, they shall recover their life after a little time, as by the space of one hour, for it is proportioned to the quality lost. And for a sure proof, if drowned Flies be put in warm ashes, they will recover their life after a little space.

The seventh herb is named of the Chaldees *Algeil*, of the Greeks *Orum*, of the Latins *Lingua canis*, of Englishmen Hound's-tongue. Put thou this herb with the heart of a young Frog and her matrix, and put them where thou wilt, and after a little time all the Dogs of the whole town shall be gathered together. And if thou shalt have the aforenamed herb under thy foremost toe, all the Dogs shall keep silence, and shall not have power to bark. And if thou shalt put the aforesaid thing in the neck of any Dog, so that he may not touch it with his mouth, he shall be turned always around about like a turning wheel, until he fall unto the ground as dead. And this hath been proved in our time.

mentioned under the name *quiritia* on p. 41; this stone must give the recipe its potency, since Pliny says that mint 'is believed to be a hindrance to generation by not allowing the genital fluids to thicken' (xx. 53. 147). The same method of reviving flies is mentioned on p. 90.

§ 9. The leaves of *Cynoglossum officinale*, hound's-tongue, contain acetamide, giving the plant a strong smell of mice, or as Gerard (1597) thought, of dog's urine. The 'matrix' is the uterus; here it probably means 'belly'. Culpeper quotes Mizaldus (Antoine Mizauld, *Alexikepus, seu auxiliaris hortus*, 1565): 'The leaves laid under the feet, will keep the dogs from barking at you.' Other methods of silencing dogs, useful no doubt to the thief, may be found below, pp. 52, 54, 61, and 56 where a reference to *lingua canis* is misunderstood.

10   The eighth herb is named of Chaldees *Mansesa*, of the Greeks *Ventosin*, of the Latins *Jusquiamus*, of Englishmen

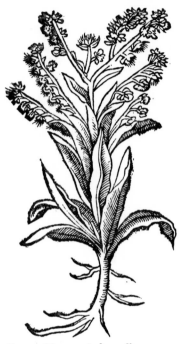

FIG. 4. *Lingua canis*, hound's-tongue.
From *Naturalia Alberti Magni* (1548)

§ 10. *Hyoscyamus niger* (henbane) was according to Turner 'named of the apothecaries *Jusquiamus*'. The plant yields the narcotic hyoscine (used by Crippen to bring about the death of his wife). Realgar is arsenic disulphide, As_2S_2, a poisonous red mineral of widespread occurrence. *Hermodactylus tuberosus* (snake's-head iris—referring to the curious purple and green flowers) is a Mediterranean plant closely related to the iris. The name *Hermodactylus* has also been applied to *Colchicum*, the 'autumn crocuses', although they are much more closely related to lilies than to crocuses. *C. autumnale* (meadow saffron, naked ladies) yields the drug colchicine, of value in the treatment of gout, and is highly poisonous. The Stockholm Medical MS. (*c.* 1400) gives a recipe for bringing about a miraculous assembly of hares, involving 'jaws of henbane in a hare's skin'; the fruit of henbane was thought to resemble a jaw with molar teeth, and by the 'doctrine of signatures' (see Introduction, p. xvii) to be a cure for toothache.

Henbane. Take thou this herb, and mix it with Realgar and *Hermodatalis*, and put them in the meat of a mad Dog, and he will die anon. And if thou shalt put the juice of it with the aforesaid things in a silver cup, it shall be broken very small. And if thou shalt mix the aforesaid thing with the blood of a young Hare and keep it in the skin of an Hare, all the Hares will be gathered there until it be removed.

The ninth herb is named of the Chaldees *Ango*, of the Greeks 11 *Amala*, of the Latins *Lilium*, of the Englishmen a Lily. If thou wilt gather this herb, the Sun being in the sign of the Lion, and wilt mix it with the juice of the Laurel, or Bay tree, and afterward thou shalt put that juice under the dung of cattle a certain time, it shall be turned into worms, of the which, if powder be made, and be put about the neck of any man, or in his clothes, he shall never sleep, nor shall not be able to sleep until it be put away. And if thou shalt put the aforesaid thing under the dung of cattle, and wilt anoint any man with the worms breeding thereof, he shall be brought anon unto a fever. And if the aforesaid thing be put in any vessel where there is Cow's milk, and be covered with the skin of any Cow of one colour, all the Kine shall lose their milk.

§ 11. *Lilium candidum*, the madonna lily, has been in cultivation since Roman times, but has never been regarded as officinal. Possibly *Convallaria majalis*, lily of the valley, is intended here; extracts of the flowers of this plant have long been used as heart stimulants. A note on laurel will be found on p. 4. The frequent references in this work to the breeding of worms under the dung of cattle appear to be a magical extension of the belief that worms were spontaneously generated from corrupting matter (belief in some form of spontaneous generation was not finally abandoned until the time of Pasteur). The qualities of the herb, mineral, or beast thus 'converted' to worms are taken to be intensified by the process. The heat of dung was certainly used in alchemy; Charles Estienne (*The Countrie Farme*, 1616, p. 457) gives one example as part of the technique for distilling the blood of a goat: 'Take the blood of a young male goat . . . let it stand and settle for some time, and then cast out the water that shall swim above: after, with a tenth or twelfth part of salt, stir it well a long time, and work them together very thoroughly; this done, put it up into a vessel well stopped and luted [sealed], and bury it in a dunghill of horsedung for the space of forty days. Afterward distil it oftentimes . . . and yet it will be better if it be set in horsedung forty days more after that it is distilled.'

12   The tenth herb is called of the Chaldees *Luperax*, of the Greeks *Esifena*, of the Latins *Viscum querci*, of Englishmen Mistletoe. And it groweth in trees, being holed through. This herb with a certain other herb, which is named *Martagon*, that is *Silphium*, or *Laserpitium* as it is written in the Almain

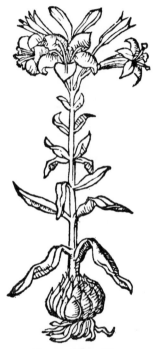

FIG. 5. *Lilium*, lily.
From *Naturalia Alberti Magni* (1548)

§ 12. The magic of *Viscum album*, mistletoe, is correlated with its evergreen and parasitic habit; in winter it is seen to flourish when its host is leafless and dormant, as though dead. Turner called the orchid *Listera ovata* (twayblade) 'martagon'; Linnaeus applied the name to *Lilium martagon*, Turk's cap lily. *Laserpitium*, according to Turner, was masterwort (*Peucedanum ostruthium*); he says 'the leaves are like unto parsley'. The plant was thought to be an antidote to poisons, and has laxative properties; as Gerard says, it is 'a great opener', which may explain the reference to locks. A more fanciful description of the way to obtain this herb is given on p. 99 in the *Marvels of the World*. The method of prophecy used here is mentioned again for the stone *selenites* on p. 28.

language, openeth all locks. And if the aforesaid things, being put together, be put in the mouth of any man, if he think of any thing, if it should happen, it is set on his heart, if not, it leapeth back from his heart. If the aforesaid thing be hanged up to a tree with the wing of a Swallow, there the birds shall be gathered together within the space of five miles. And this last was proved in my time.

The eleventh herb is named of the Chaldees *Isiphilon*, of the Greeks *Orgelon*, of the Latins *Centaurea*, of Englishmen Centaury. Witches say that this herb hath a marvellous virtue, for if it be joined with the blood of a female Lapwing, or Black Plover, and be put with oil in a lamp, all they that compass it about shall believe themselves to be witches, so that one shall believe of another that his head is in heaven and his feet in the earth. And if the aforesaid thing be put in the fire when the stars shine it shall appear that the stars run one against another, and fight. And if the aforesaid plaster be put to the nostrils of any man, he shall flee away sharply, through fear that he shall have. And this hath been proved.

The twelfth herb is named of the Chaldees *Colorio*, or 14

§ 13. Centaury is *Centaurium erythrea*, a pink flower of pastures, named by Hippocrates for Chiron the Centaur, who had wide knowledge of herbs; it is a bitter-tasting plant, thought to have tonic properties and to be good against bleeding and fevers. *Centaurea cyanus* is a blue-flowered weed of cultivation (cornflower). Here the smoke of the burning herb is apparently thought to have hallucinogenic properties; there are many similar recipes in the *Marvels of the World* in the section from the *Book of Fires* by Marcus Grecus, pp. 97 ff. below. 'Witches' translates the Latin *Magi* (see Introduction, p. xxxix). A note on the lapwing will be found on p. 56.

§ 14. Sage (*Salvia officinalis*) is thought of now as a culinary herb, but the Elizabethans, taking a hint from the name, found medicinal uses for it:

> In Latin, *Salvia*, takes the name of safety,
> In English, *Sage*, is rather wise than crafty:
> Sith then the name betokens wise and saving,
> We count it nature's friend, and worth the having

(from *The English Doctor*, 1609, sig. B.6, a translation by Sir John Harington of the *Regimen Sanitatis Salerni*). Culpeper thought that it was 'of excellent use to help the memory, warming and quickening the senses'. It was said by Pliny to cure snakebite. See p. 60 for a note on the 'Black Mack or Ousel'.

Coloricon, of the Greeks *Clamor,* of the Latins commonly *Salvia,* of Englishmen Sage. This herb, being putrefied under dung of cattle in a glassen vessel, bringeth forth a certain worm, or bird having a tail after the fashion of that bird called a Black Mack or Ousel, with whose blood, if any man be touched on the breast, he shall lose his sense or feeling the space of fifteen

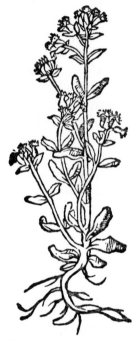

FIG. 6. *Centaurea,* centaury.
From *Naturalia Alberti Magni* (1548)

days and more. And if the aforesaid Serpent be burned, and the ashes of it put in the fire, anon shall there be a rainbow, with an horrible thunder. And if the aforesaid ashes be put in a lamp, and be kindled, it shall appear that all the house is full of Serpents, and this hath been proved of men of late time.

15   The thirteenth herb is named of the Chaldees *Olphanas,* of

§ 15. Vervain is *Verbena officinalis* (see note, p. 21). Its Welsh name is *llysiau'r*

the Greeks *Hiliorion*, of the Latins *Verbena*, of the Englishmen Vervain. This herb (as Witches say) gathered, the Sun being in the sign of the Ram, and put with grain or corn of Peony of one year old, healeth them that be sick of the falling sickness. And if it be put in a fat ground, after eight weeks worms shall

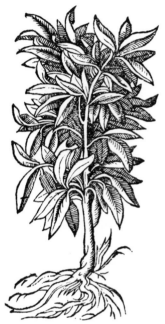

FIG. 7. *Salvia*, sage.
From *Naturalia Alberti Magni* (1548)

be engendered, which, if they shall touch any man, he shall die anon. And if the aforesaid thing be put in a Dove house or a Culver house, all the Doves or Culvers shall be gathered

budol, 'herb of enchantment', and according to the Stockholm Medical MS. (*c.* 1400), it is powerful against 'the devil of hell'; the 'falling sickness' (epilepsy) was often thought to be the result of possession by devils. Peony is *Paeonia officinalis*, a name derived from Paeon, physician to the gods of Olympus. A 'fat ground' is fertile soil; for a note on the effect of worms, see p. 11. The sympathetic magic used to gather culvers (doves) may be explained by the other names given to vervain on p. 22.

together there. And if the powder of them be put in the Sun, it shall appear that the Sun is blue. If the powder be put in a place where men dwell, or lie between two lovers, anon there is made strife or malice between them.

16   The fourteenth herb is named of the Chaldees *Celayos*, of the Greeks *Casini*, of the Latins *Melissophyllum*, of Englishmen Smallage; of the which herb Macer Floridus maketh mention. This herb, gathered green, and casten with the juice of the Cypress tree of one year, put in gruel, maketh the gruel to appear full of worms, and maketh the bearer to be gentle and gracious, and to vanquish his adversaries. And if the aforesaid herb be bounden to an Ox's neck, he will follow thee whither-soever thou wilt go.

17   The fifteenth herb is named of the Chaldees *Glerisa*, of the Greeks *Isaphinus*, of the Latins *Rosa*, of Englishmen a Rose. And it is an herb whose flower is very well known. Take the grain or corn of it, and the corn of Mustard seed and the foot of a Weasel; hang up these in a tree, and it will not bear fruit after. And if the aforesaid thing be put about a net, fishes will

§ 16. *Melissophyllum* is a name used by Pliny and Virgil, meaning 'bee plant'; it was applied by Linnaeus to *Melittis melissophyllum*, an aromatic herb known as 'bastard balm' to distinguish it from the related plant *Melissa officinalis* (balm), which may be the herb intended here. Aemilius Macer wrote on plants in the first century B.C., and a herbalist whose real name was probably Odo took the pseudonym 'Macer Floridus' in about the tenth century; the writer referred to here is probably the medieval herbalist, though he does not in fact report these properties of *melissophyllum*. 'Smallage', according to Turner, is *Apium graveolens* (wild celery). A more plausible way of making food appear full of worms is suggested by Jean Baptista Porta: 'If you cut Harp-strings small, and strew them on hot flesh, the heat will twist them, and they will move like worms' (*Natural Magic*, trans. 1658, reprinted New York, 1957; p. 327).

§ 17. The rose has been in cultivation since Roman times, but has never been regarded as officinal. The properties attributed to it are not consistent, as it is credited with the power both of inducing sterility and of restoring life. *Magaris* has not been identified, though it may be a reference to pearls (*margaritae*), which can lose 'life' or lustre. Olive oil and powdered sulphur ('quick brim-stone') are inflammable; this recipe, and the one following, are clearly from the *Book of Fires* as are those recipes in the *Marvels of the World* (see p. 97) which deal with supposed hallucinogens absorbed through their smoke ('put in a lamp').

gather together there. And if *Magaris* shall be dead and be put in the aforesaid commixion half a day, it shall recover the life, although it be not forthwith yet gotten. And if the aforesaid powder be put in a lamp, and after be kindled, all men shall appear black as the devil. And if the aforesaid powder be mixed with oil of the Olive tree and with quick Brimstone,

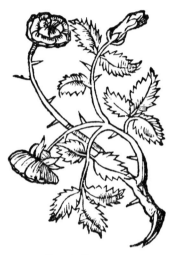

FIG. 8. *Rosa*, rose.
From *Naturalia Alberti Magni* (1548)

and the house anointed with it, the sun shining, it shall appear all inflamed.

The sixteenth herb is called of the Chaldees *Carturlin*, of the Greeks *Pentaphyllon*, of the Latins *Serpentina*, in English Snake's-grass. This herb is well enough known with us. This herb put in the ground, with the leaf of the Three-leaved Grass, engendereth red and green Serpents, of which if powder

§ 18. The Greek name here is genuine, but must have been substituted by the translator, as the Latin texts have *quinquefolium*, a Latin synonym for *serpentina*. *Fritillaria meleagris*, chequered lily, is called snake's head and five-leaved grass. Snake's-grass is another name for *Achillea millefolium*, see note, p. 5, and *pentaphyllon* is properly *Potentilla reptans*, cinquefoil, see note, p. 20. Three-leaved grass is clover (*Trifolium* sp.); Pliny (xxi. 88. 152) says that serpents will not venture into clover.

　　　　　　　　　　E

be made, and be put in a burning lamp, there shall appear abundance of Serpents. And if it be put under the head of any man, from thenceforth he shall not dream of himself.

19   The manner of working all these aforenamed things, that the effect may be good in their planets, is in their hours, and days.

20   There be seven herbs that have great virtues, after the mind of Alexander the Emperor, and they have these virtues of the influence of the planets. And therefore, every one of them taketh their virtue from the higher natural powers.

21   The first is the herb of the planet Saturn, which is called *Daffodillus*, Daffodilly. The juice of it is good against the pain of the reins, and legs; let them that suffer pain of the bladder, eat it, the root of it being a little boiled. And if men possessed with evil spirits, or mad men, bear it in a clean napkin, they be delivered from their disease. And it suffereth not a devil in the house. And if children that breed their teeth, bear it about them, they shall breed them without pain. And it is good that a man bear with him a root of it in the night for he shall not fear, nor be hurt of other.

22   The second is the herb of the Sun, which is called *Poly-*

§ 19. For a further discussion of the 'hours and days' of astrological influence, see pp. 62 ff.

§ 20. The seven planetary herbs and their properties in this section have more frequently been ascribed to Alexius Affricus or Flaccus Africanus than to Alexander the Great. The properties claimed for the herbs are more medical than magical, and are for the greater part derived either from the qualities associated with the planets themselves, or from a connection with the parts of the body over which the planet held dominion; see the section on the seven planets, pp. 65 ff.

§ 21. The wild yellow daffodil is *Narcissus pseudonarcissus*. The English names come via the medieval Latin *affodilus* from the Greek *asphodelus*, the flowers that grew in the meadows of the underworld. Turner calls *Asphodelus ramosus* 'white daffodil', distinguishing it from *N. pseudonarcissus*, 'yellow daffodil'. The reins are the kidneys. The phrase 'mad men' is a translation of the Latin *melancholici*; Saturn is of 'complexion melancholic' (see p. 66). Of the power against devils, Pliny says 'there is a tradition that if asphodel be planted before the gate of a country house it keeps away the evil influences of sorcery' (xxi. 67. 108).

§ 22. *Polygonum aviculare* is a common astringent herb which Culpeper says 'is

gonum, or *Corrigiola.* This herb taketh the name of the Sun, for it engendereth greatly, and so this herb worketh many ways. Other hath called this herb *Alchone,* which is the house of the Sun. This herb healeth the passions and griefs of the heart and the stomach. He that toucheth this herb hath a virtue of his sign, or planet. If any man drink the juice of it, it maketh him to do often the act of generation. And if any man bear the root of it, it healeth the grief of the eyes. And if he bear it with him before he have any grief, there shall come to him no grief of his eyes. It helpeth also them that be vexed with the frenzy, if they bear it with them in their breast. It helpeth also them that are diseased with an impostume in the lungs, and maketh them to have a good breath; and it availeth also to the flux of melancholious blood.

The third is the herb of the Moon, which is called *Chyno-* 23 *states.* The juice of it purgeth the pains of the stomach, and breast plates. The virtue of it declareth that it is the herb of the Moon. The flower of this herb purgeth great spleens and healeth them, because this herb increaseth and decreaseth as the Moon. It is good against the sickness of the eyes, and maketh a sharp sight. And it is good against the blood of the eyes. If thou put the root of it brayed upon the eye, it will make the eye marvellous clear, because the light of the eyes has *propinquatum mysticum* [a mystical affinity] with the substance of the Moon.

under the dominion of Saturn; yet some hold of the Sun'. According to Turner, in French it is called 'la corrigiole', but *Corrigiola litoralis* is a quite unrelated and much less common plant. The reference to *Alchone* is obscure; the astrological house of the sun is *Leo.* Most of the magic of this plant comes by sympathetic association with the life-giving sun. An impostume is an abscess, and 'melancholious' blood is dark, or venous blood.

§ 23. This may be chickweed (*Stellaria media*), which is called 'moonwort' or 'moonflower' in Yorkshire; however, as the author says, the properties given could apply to any herb held to be under the dominion of the moon. The spleen was believed to be the source of the melancholy humour, and was thought to increase and decrease with the moon. 'Brayed' means 'powdered'. The 'swine pox' here and elsewhere is a mistranslation of the Latin word *scrophula,* scrofula, a disease also known as the 'king's evil', involving swelling of the glands.

It is also good to them that have an evil stomach or which cannot digest their meat, by drinking the juice of it. Moreover it is good to them that have the swine pox.

24   The fourth herb is called *Arnoglossus*, Plantain. The root of this herb is marvellous good against the pain of the head, because the sign of the Ram is supposed to be the house of the planet Mars, which is the head of the whole world. It is good also against evil customs of man's stones, and rotten and filthy boils, because his house is the sign *Scorpio*, [and] because a part of it holdeth *Sperma*, that is the seed, which cometh from the stones, whereof all living things be engendered, and formed. Also the juice of it is good to them that be sick of the perilous flux, with excoriation or razing of the bowels, continual torments, and some blood issuing forth. And it purgeth them that drink it from the sickness of the flux of blood, or haemorrhoids, and of the disease of the stomach.

25   The fifth is the herb of the planet Mercury, which is named *Pentaphyllon*, in English Cinquefoil or the Five-leaved herb; of others *Pentadactylus*, of others *Sepedeclinans*, of certain *Calipendalo*. The root of this herb brayed and made in a plaster,

§ 24. Probably the two species *Plantago major* and *P. media* were not clearly distinguished, though the softly and finely hairy leaves of the latter are more like a 'lamb's tongue' (*arnoglossus*) than the smooth leaves of *P. major*. Culpeper says 'Mizaldus and others hold this to be a herb of Mars; the truth is it is under the command of Venus, and cures the head by antipathy to Mars and the privities by sympathy to Venus'—a good example of having it both ways. Here it is explained in terms of the two signs of the zodiac which are associated with Mars; the Ram (*Aries*), which has dominion over the head, and *Scorpio*, which controls the sexual organs, here specifically the testicles ('stones'). The whole phrase 'them that be sick of the perilous flux . . . some blood issuing forth' is Elyot's translation of the word found in the Latin text, *dysenterici*, 'those who have dysentery'.

§ 25. The names given here for *Potentilla reptans* refer to its palmate leaves with five leaflets (though Turner's name, *quinquefolium*, is not mentioned), its liking for hedge-banks (*sepedeclinans*), and the modest beauty of the plant (*calipendalo*). It was esteemed in Europe as an apotropaic herb, but Reginald Scot (*The Discoverie of Witchcraft*, 1584) is contemptuous of its use to repel witches. The properties here are derived from the belief that Mercury had influence over eloquence (see p. 72). 'Stone' refers to gall-stones, and 'letteth' means 'stoppeth'.

healeth wounds and hardness. Moreover, it putteth away quickly the swine pox, if the juice of it be drunken with water. It healeth also the passions or griefs of the breast, if the juice of it be drunken. It putteth away also the toothache. And if the juice of it be holden in the mouth, it healeth all the griefs of the mouth, and if any man bear it with him, it giveth work and help. Moreover if any man will ask any thing of a king or prince, it giveth abundance of eloquence, if he have it with him, and he shall obtain it that he desireth. It is also good to have the juice of it, for the grief of the stone, and the sickness which letteth a man that [he] can not piss.

The sixth is the herb of the planet Jupiter, and is named 26 *Acharonis*, of certain *Jusquiamus*, Henbane. The root of it, put upon botches, healeth them, and keepeth the place from an inflammation of blood. If any man shall bear it before the grief come upon him he shall never have a botch. The root of it also is profitable against the gout in the feet when it is brayed, and put upon the place that suffereth the pain or grief. And it worketh by virtue of those signs, which have feet, and look upon the feet. And if the juice of it be drunken with honey, or with wine and honey sodden together, it is profitable against the griefs of the liver, and all his passions, because Jupiter holdeth the liver. Likewise, it is profitable to them that would do often the act of generation; and to them that desire to be loved of women, it is good that they bear it with them, for it maketh the bearers pleasant and delectable.

The seventh is the herb of the planet Venus, and is called 27

§ 26. *Hyoscyamus niger*, henbane, is a narcotic herb (see note, p. 10) which proved less dangerous in the hands of medieval physicians than the related *Atropa belladonna*, deadly nightshade, and achieved a wide reputation, especially as a sedative. 'Botches' are boils. Pliny (xxvi. 64. 100) reports the beneficial effect of henbane on gout, explained here astrologically; Jupiter is associated with the sign *Pisces*, which in turn has dominion over the feet. 'Sodden' means 'boiled'. The Stockholm Medical MS. (*c.* 1400) says: 'If thou shouldst go amongst women' carrying henbane, 'it shall them make to love thee all.'

§ 27. 'Verbena' is a name used by Pliny for a plant used in religious ceremonies; Turner says it was called *Peristerion* in Greek. *Hierobotane* is mentioned by both Dioscorides and Pliny as a sacred herb. In the Middle Ages they were both

Peristerion, of some *Hierobotane, id est Herba columbaria*, and *Verbena*, Vervain. The root of this herb put upon the neck healeth the swine pox, impostumes behind the ears, and botches of the neck, and such as can not keep their water. It healeth also cuts, and swelling of the tewel, or fundament, pro-ceeding of an inflammation which groweth in the fundament;

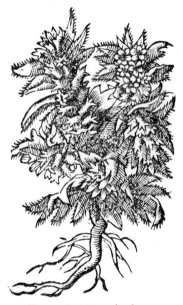

FIG. 9. *Jusquiamus*, henbane.
From *Naturalia Alberti Magni* (1548)

and the haemorrhoids. If the juice of it be drunken with honey and water sodden, it dissolveth those things which are in the lungs or lights. And it maketh a good breath, for it saveth and keepeth the lungs and the lights. It is also of great strength in

assumed to be vervain (*Verbena officinalis*). Gerard says 'Many old wives' tales are written of Vervain . . . I am not willing to trouble your ears with such trifles', and that some physicians use it for the plague, but 'it is no remedy at all'. Nevertheless, John Morley in his *Essay . . . on the King's Evil* (1767) regards the plant as a sovereign remedy for scrofula. *Herba columbaria* is a different plant, *Aquilegia vulgaris*, columbine. Botches and impostumes are boils. The tewel, as the text explains, is the 'fundament' or anus.

venereal pastimes, that is, the act of generation. If any man put
it in his house or vineyard, or in the ground, he shall have
abundantly revenues, or yearly profits; moreover the root of it is
good to all them which will plant vineyards or trees. And
infants bearing it shall be very apt to learn, and loving learning,

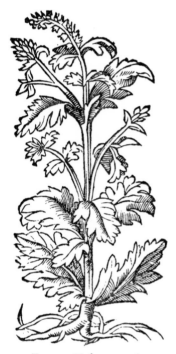

FIG. 10. *Verbena*, vervain.
From *Naturalia Alberti Magni* (1548)

and they shall be glad and joyous. It is also profitable, being
put in purgations, and it putteth aback devils.

   Yet this is to be marked, that these herbs be gathered from 28
the twenty-third day of the Moon until the thirtieth day,

§ 28. The translator was confused by a Latin text which is far from clear. The
passage probably means that the herbs are to be gathered each day in the hour
governed by Mercury (see p. 64).

beginning the gathering of them from the sign *Mercurius*, by the space of a whole hour, and in gathering make mention of the passion or grief, and the name of the thing for the which thou dost gather it. Notwithstanding, lay the same herb upon Wheat, or Barley, and use it afterward to thy need.

Here beginneth the Second Book, of the Virtues of Certain Stones

Now because I have spoken before of the virtues of certain 1
herbs, now in this present chapter I will speak of certain stones,
their effects and marvellous operations.

Magnes, the Loadstone

Ophthalmus	*Onyx*
Peridonius	*Selenites*
Topazos	*Medius*
Memphites	*Asbestos*
Adamas, Diamond	*Achates*
Alectoria	*Amandinus*
Amethystus	*Beryllus*
Chelonites	*Corallus*
Crystallus	*Heliotropium*
Hephaestites	*Chalcedonius*
Chelidonius	*Gagatronica*
Hyaenia	*Schistos*
Kabrates	*Chrysolithus*
Gerachidem	*Nicomar*
Quiritia	*Radaim*
Liparea	*Virites*
Lazuli	*Smaragdus*
Iris	*Chalazia*
Gagates	*Draconites*
Aetites	*Hephaestites*

§ 1. The names of these stones are adopted from Pliny, where possible; those
which cannot be identified with certainty, or which Pliny does not mention,
are taken from Wyckoff's translation of the alphabetical lapidary in the
Mineralia of Albertus Magnus, the immediate source of this section. The names
of a number of stones were so corrupted that the originals in Albertus Magnus
could be traced only by finding the stone with identical properties ascribed to it.

| *Hyacinthus* | *Orites* |
| *Sappirus* | *Samius* |

2   If thou wilt know whether thy wife
                     be chaste, or no.

Take the stone which is called *Magnes*, in English the Load⁄
stone. It is of sad blue colour, and it is found in the sea of
India, sometimes in parts of Almany, in the province which is
called East France. Lay this stone under the head of a wife, and
if she be chaste, she will embrace her husband; if she be not
chaste, she will fall anon forth of the bed. Moreover, if this
stone be put brayed and scattered upon coals, in four corners
of the house, they that be sleeping shall flee the house, and
leave all.

3   If thou wilt be made invisible.

Take the stone which is called *Ophthalmus*, and wrap it in the
leaf of the Laurel, or Bay tree; and it is called *Lapis Obtalmicus*,
whose colour is not named, for it is of many colours. And it is
of such virtue, that it blindeth the sights of them that stand

§ 2. *Magnes* is magnetite (magnetic iron oxide, Fe_3O_4). Wyckoff remarks 'the
swift "embrace" of magnetite and iron—for which William Gilbert in 1600
used the term *coitus*—obviously suggested its use as a love charm'. She further
remarks of the powder scattered upon coals that 'something other than magnetite
must be meant—perhaps bitumen, or perhaps some drug "from Magnesia"'
(there were several places called 'Magnesia' in antiquity). 'Sad blue colour'
may be explained by Elyot's translation of the Latin word *ferrugineus* as 'rust
of iron, a muddy colour, some call it sad [dark] blue'. Almany is Germany,
and 'East France' (*francia orientalis* in the Latin text) is a corruption of *Franconia*,
mentioned by Albertus Magnus in this context. *Franconia* was central Germany,
the modern province of Franken. The Latin text, following Albertus Magnus,
goes on to reveal the point of the last property: 'and then the thieves steal
whatever they want'.

§ 3. *Ophthalmus* is precious opal, an impure form of silica (SiO_2) which shows
a play of colours as light strikes it at different angles. Constantius is probably
Constantinus Africanus (*c.* 1015–87), and he was made 'invisible' because the
bright colours of the stone dazzled the bystanders. The 'Laurel, or Bay tree' is
Laurus nobilis, see note, p. 4.

about. Constantius carrying this in his hand, was made invisible by it.

> If thou wilt provoke sorrow, fear, 4
> terrible fantasies, and debate.

Take the stone which is called *Onyx*, which is of black colour. And the kind is best which is full of white veins. And it cometh from India, unto Araby, and if it be hanged upon the neck, or finger, it stirreth up anon sorrow or heaviness in a man, and terrors, and also debate. And this hath been proved by men of late time.

> If thou wilt burn any man's 5
> hands without fire.

Take the stone which is called *Peridonius*, which is of yellow colour, which if it be hanged upon the neck of any man, it healeth *Areticum*. And also if this stone be gripped straitly, it burneth the hand anon, and therefore it must be touched lightly, and gently.

> If thou wilt kindle the mind of any man 6
> to joys, and make his wit sharp.

Take the stone which is called *Selenites*. It groweth in the bosom of a snail of India, called Tortoise, and there is of divers

§ 4. Onyx is chalcedony (a form of silica, SiO_2) with contrastingly coloured layers; it is a hard stone used for cameos. Onyx marble is a banded travertine (impure limestone, $CaCO_3$), and is softer. The first of several claims of 'recent proof' in this section is made here; Albertus Magnus makes this claim only for *Alectoria, Corallus* and *Hephaestites*.

§ 5. *Peridonius* is peridot, a dark green form of olivine ($2(Mg,Fe)O.SiO_2$). The properties given, however, refer to pyrites, which appears again, mis-spelled differently as *virites*, and also under *hephaestites*. 'Gripped straitly' means tightly; Wyckoff remarks that 'pyrites on weathering, produces sulphuric acid, that would irritate the hands'. *Areticum*, which appears as *arteticam* in less corrupted Latin texts, is apparently a misprint for the late Latin *arterica*, 'bronchitis'.

§ 6. *Selenites, silenites* according to Albertus Magnus, is selenite, a crystalline

kinds of it, of white, red, and purple colour. Others say that
it is green, and found in the parts of Persia. And also old
Philosophers say, if it be tasted, it giveth knowledge of certain
things to come. If it be put under the tongue, specially in the
first [day of the] Moon, it hath a virtue only for an hour. Therefore being in the tenth day of the Moon, it hath this virtue in
the first or tenth hour. The method of divination is this: when
it is under the tongue, if our thought be of any business,
whether it ought to be or no, if it ought to be, it is fixed steadfastly to the heart, so that it may not be plucked away, if not,
the heart leapeth aback from it. Also Philosophers have said
that it healeth phthisics, and weak men.

7   If thou wilt that seething water come forth anon,
                   after thou hast put in thy hand.

Take the stone which is called *Topazos* from the isle Topazis,
or because it showeth a similitude of gold. And there be two
kinds of it; one is utterly like gold and this is more precious,

form of gypsum ($CaSO_4$). The properties, however, refer to *chelonites* (see p.
34) which Pliny says 'comes from the eye of an Indian tortoise'. The English
translator had some difficulty with this passage, apparently because his Latin
text was garbled; our version follows Wyckoff, but the sense is still not clear;
it may be a confused reference to the astrological 'hours of the day'—see pp. 62
ff. 'It is fixed steadfastly to the heart' is translated from Albertus Magnus,
by Wyckoff, as 'the heart is seized by a firm conviction'. 'Phthisics' are
consumptives.

§ 7. *Topazos* in Pliny is a green stone (olivine, $2(Mg,Fe)O.SiO_2$) from the
island of Topazos. Later the name became transferred to a yellow ('the colour
of saffron') transparent stone (topaz, $Al_2F_2SiO_4$). Here it is confused with
hephaestites, pyrites, to which the properties refer. Albertus Magnus says of
'*topasion*' that 'if it is put into boiling water it makes the water stop bubbling,
so that soon the hand can be put in to take it out', and Wyckoff remarks that
'any cold stone would of course stop the boiling'. She also points out that
Pliny's phrase *limam sentit*, 'feels the file' (olivine is fairly soft), is miscopied or
misread by Marbod (see p. xxxv) as *lunam sentire putatur*, 'is thought to feel the
moon', which accounts for the reference here to 'lunatic passion'. *Emothoicam* is
a corruption of *haemorrhoidam*, haemorrhoids, and *stimaticam* (which does not
appear in Albertus) probably means 'a state of excitement'.

the other kind is of the colour of saffron, of brighter colour than gold is, and this is more profitable. It hath been proved, in our time, that if it be put in seething water it maketh it to run over, but if thou put thy hand in it, the water is drawn out anon, and one of our brethren did this at Paris. It is good also against *emothoicam et stimaticam,* or lunatic passion or grief.

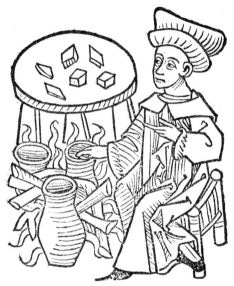

FIG. 11. *Topazos.*
From the *Hortus Sanitatis* (1491)

If thou wilt pluck off the skin of thine,   **8**
or another man's hand.

Take the stone which is called *Medius,* of the region Media, in the which the people dwelling are called Medes. And there be two kinds of it, black and green. It is said of old Philosophers

§ 8. *Medius,* Wyckoff suggests, was probably a mixture of impure metallic sulphates, also known as atramentum, produced by the weathering of copper pyrites ($CuFeS_2$). Some free sulphuric acid might well be present in such a mixture. 'Resolved' means 'dissolved'. The Medes were inhabitants of the northern part of the Babylonian Empire (the north-western part of modern Iran).

and also of Philosophers being in this time, if the black be broken, and resolved in hot water, if any man wash his hands in that water, the skin of his hands shall be plucked off anon. Philosophers say also, that it is good against the gout, and blindness of the eyes, and it nourisheth hurt and weak eyes.

9

If thou wilt that a man suffer no pain, nor be tormented.

Take the stone which is called *Memphites*, of the city which is called Memphis, and it is a stone of such virtue as Aaron and Hermes say: if it be broken, and mixed with water, and given to him to drink, which should be burned, or suffer any torments, that drink induceth so great unableness to feel, that he that suffereth, feeleth neither pain nor tormenting.

10

If thou wilt make a fire continually unable to be quenched or put out.

Take the stone which is called *Asbestos*, and it is of the colour of Iron, and there is found very much of it in Arabia. If that stone be kindled or inflamed, it may never be put out, or quenched, because it hath the nature of the first feathers of

§ 9. 'Memphis stone' may have been dolomite ($CaCO_3.MgCO_3$) but the 'properties' given are more likely to apply to a vegetable drug. For notes on Aaron and Hermes, see the Introduction, pp. xxxvi and xxxix.

§ 10. *Asbestos, abeston* in Albertus Magnus, is asbestos (fibrous amphibole, a complex silicate of calcium, magnesium, and iron). The salamander mentioned here is the legendary beast which, according to Paracelsus, was the spirit of the Aristotelian element, fire; it was supposed to live in fire in much the same way as a fish, for instance, lives in water. Albertus Magnus (*Meteora*, iv. 3. 17) says: 'That . . . which in common speech is called "salamander's down" . . . is like cloth woven out of wool.' If it were in fact woven from asbestos, it could have been used as a wick, and would have burned without being consumed; this may have been the secret of ever-burning lamps in temples.

the Salamander, by reason of moisty fatness, which nourisheth the fire kindled in it.

If thou wilt overcome thy enemies.   11

Take the stone which is called *Adamas*, in English speech a Diamond, and it is of shining colour, and very hard, in so much that it cannot be broken, but by the blood of a Goat, and it groweth in Arabia, or in Cyprus. And if it be bounden to

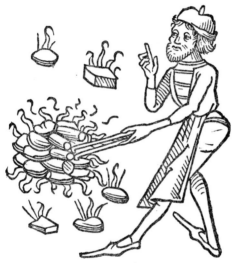

FIG. 12. *Asbestos.*
From the *Hortus Sanitatis* (1491)

the left side, it is good against enemies, madness, wild beasts, venomous beasts, and cruel men, and against chiding and brawling, and against venom, and invasion of fantasies. And some call it *Diamas*.

§ 11. Diamond, a crystalline form of carbon, is clearly described here, although the properties given are purely magical. Of the phrase 'cannot be broken, but by the blood of a goat', Wyckoff remarks: 'This comes from Pliny, and it is difficult to imagine any basis for it unless Pliny took literally some Alexandrian "cover name" for a compound used in grinding and polishing gems.'

12   If thou wilt eschew all perils and all terrible
                things, and have a strong heart.

Take the stone which is called *Achates*, and it is black, and
hath white veins. There is another of the same kind, like to
white colour. And the third groweth in a certain Isle; it has
black veins, and that maketh to overcome perils, and give
strength to the heart, and maketh a man mighty, pleasant,
delectable, and helpeth against adversities.

13   If thou desire to obtain any
                        thing from any man.

Take the stone which is called *Alectoria*, and it is a stone of a
Cock, and it is white as the Crystal, and it is drawn out of the
Cock's gizzard, or maw, after that he hath been gelded more
than four years, and it is of the greatness of a bean. It maketh
the belly pleasant and steadfast, and, put under the tongue, it
quencheth thirst. And this last hath been proved in our time,
and I perceived it quickly.

14   If thou wilt overcome beasts, and interpret or expound
            all dreams and prophesy of things to come.

Take the stone which is called *Amandinus*. It is of divers
colours. It putteth out all poison, and maketh a man to over⁄

§ 12. *Achates, agathes* in Albertus Magnus, is agate (banded chalcedony, a form
of silica, SiO_2). The 'certain isle' is, according to Albertus Magnus, the island
of Crete; at some stage *Creta* was transposed to *certa* in the Latin text.

§ 13. Albertus Magnus (*Animalia*, xxiii. 46) says: 'A capon is a cock that is
castrated and effeminate . . . It is said that after six years a stone named *electorius*
grows in its liver, and from that time onwards the capon does not drink. And
therefore a man who wears this stone is said not to get thirsty.' Thus the 'cock⁄
stone' could be a tumour, or perhaps an unusually transparent pebble from the
gizzard. As Wyckoff remarks, sucking a pebble does keep the mouth from
getting dry. Albertus Magnus also says that the properties given are 'a matter
of experience' which is rendered here as having been 'proved'.

§ 14. '*Amandinus*' is possibly a corruption of *amiantus*, mentioned by Pliny, and
said to afford protection against magicians' spells. To 'assoil' is to 'resolve' or

come his adversaries, and giveth prophesying, and the interpretation of all dreams, and maketh a man to understand dark
questions, hard to be understood or assoiled.

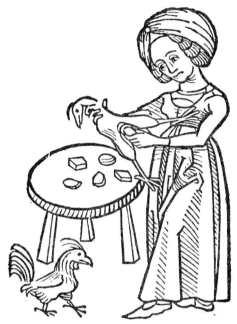

FIG. 13. *Alectoria.*
From the *Hortus Sanitatis* (1491)

If thou wilt have good understanding of things that may be   15
felt, and that thou may not be made drunken.

Take the stone which is called *Amethystus*, and it is of purple
colour, and the best is found in India. And it is good against

to 'solve'; the whole phrase ('dark questions . . .') is an explanation of the word
enigmata in the Latin text.

§ 15. Amethyst is a quartz (crystalline silica, SiO_2) gem, wine-coloured due
to traces of manganese. Pliny supposed that 'amethystus' meant 'not drunken'
and tried to justify this by referring to the colour of the stone, but he was
contemptuous of the belief (attributed by Albertus Magnus to the unidentified
'Aaron') that it prevents drunkenness. The phrase 'things that may be felt' in

drunkenness, and giveth good understanding in things that may be understood.

16   *If thou wilt overcome thy enemies,*
                          and flee debate.

Take the stone which is called *Beryllus*. It is of pale colour and may be seen through as water. Bear it about with thee, and thou shalt overcome all debate, and shalt drive away thy enemies, and it maketh thy enemy meek. It causeth a man to be well mannered, as Aaron saith. It giveth also good under/standing.

17   *If thou wilt forejudge, or conjecture*
                          of things to come.

Take the stone which is called *Chelonites*. It is of purple, and divers other colours, and it is found in the head of the Snail. If any man will bear this stone under his tongue, he shall fore/judge, and prophesy of things to come. But notwithstanding, it is said to have this power only on the first day of the [lunar] month, when the Moon is rising and waxing, and again on the twenty/ninth day when the Moon is waning. So meaneth Aaron in the book of virtues of herbs, and stones.

the heading is a translation of the obscure word *sensibus*, in the Latin text, probably a corruption of the expression which appears later, *scibilibus*, 'things that may be understood'.

§ 16. Beryl ($BeO.Al_2O_3.6SiO_2$) is a green gemstone found as hexagonal prisms. Pliny describes the colour as 'the pure green of the sea', and Wyckoff points out that medieval writers took this to mean 'as clear as water'.

§ 17. *Chelonites*, according to Pliny, 'is the eye of the Indian tortoise' (xxxvii. 56. 155). Albertus Magnus, who calls it *celontes*, states that 'it is said to be found in the body of a shellfish; for some very large shellfish have dwellings that gleam with a pearly lustre', and, as Wyckoff remarks, 'he is plainly describing mother/of/pearl'. The translator, misled by a misprint in his Latin text, left much of this passage confused; our version follows Wyckoff.

> If thou wilt pacify tempests   18
> and go over floods.

Take the stone which is called *Corallus*, Coral, and some be
red and some white. And it hath been proved that it stemmeth
anon blood, putteth away the foolishness of him that beareth it,
and giveth wisdom. And this hath been proved of certain men
in our time. And it is good against tempests, and perils of
floods.

> If thou wilt kindle fire.   19

Take the Crystal stone, and put it nigh under the circle of the
Sun, that is to say, against the Sun, and put it nigh any thing
that may be burned, and incontinently the heat of the Sun
shining will set it afire. And if it be drunk with honey, it
increaseth milk.

> If thou wilt that the Sun appear of   20
> bloody colour.

Take the stone which is called *Heliotropium*. It is green like to
the precious stone called the Emerald. And it is sprinkled with

§ 18. Coral was supposed by Pliny to be a plant that grows in the sea and is
changed to stone when brought up into the air. Its use for stanching bleeding
is sympathetic magic suggested by the blood-red colour of the commonest form
of the stone. Albertus Magnus says it is good against epilepsy and that the
properties given have been 'found by experience'.

§ 19. Rock crystal is clear, colourless quartz (SiO_2). It would obviously be a
suitable material from which to make a 'burning glass'; and no doubt the
honey would do a nursing mother good. There are two crystal balls in the
mineral collection of Sir Hans Sloane (1660-1753) in the British Museum
(Natural History), one smooth and one faceted. Sloane comments in his
manuscript catalogue that they were to cool the hands of patients during fever.

§ 20. Heliotrope or bloodstone is a variety of chalcedony (a form of silica,
SiO_2), and its colour is dark green, streaked with red. The name 'Babylonian
gems' stems from Pliny's account (xxxvii. 60. 165) of a claim by the Magi
(Babylonian priest-magicians), which he says is 'most blatant effrontery', that
when the stone is combined with the plant of the same name (*Heliotropium
europaeum*, see note, p. 4) it confers invisibility. Pliny also says that the stone,
put into a vessel of water, 'in reflecting the sunlight it changes it into the colour

bloody drops. The necromancers call it *Gemma Babylonica*, the precious stone of Babylon, by the proper name. But if it be anointed with the juice of an herb of the same name, and be put in a vessel full of water, it maketh the Sun to seem of bloody colour, as if the eclipse were seen. The cause of this is for it maketh all the water to bubble up unto a little cloud, which, making the air thick, letteth the Sun to be seen, but as it were red, in a thick colour. A little after the cloud goeth away, by dropping down like dew, as it were by drops of rain. This also borne about maketh a man of good fame, whole and of long life. It is said of old Philosophers that a man anointed with an herb of this name, as we have said before, excelleth with virtue. And *Heliotropium* is found oftentimes in Cyprus and India.

21   If thou wilt make seething water to be cold,
               which standeth upon the fire.

Take the stone which is called *Hephaestites*, which, put in water against the eye of the Sun, putteth forth fiery beams of the Sun. And it is said of old and new Philosophers, if it be put in seething water, the bubbling up or seething will soon cease, and a little after, it will wax cold. And it is a shining and ruddy stone.

22   If thou wilt eschew illusions and fantasies
            and overcome all causes or matters.

Take the stone which is called *Chalcedonius*, and it is pale, brown of colour, and somewhat dark. If this be pierced with

of blood', but as Wyckoff points out, Albertus Magnus (who calls it *eliotropia*) appears to think that some sort of chemical reaction takes place causing effervescence, followed by the formation of a precipitate, perhaps. 'Letteth' is used in the sense 'preventeth'.

§ 21. *Hephaestites*, Albertus Magnus's *epistrites*, is pyrites (iron sulphide, FeS_2), a brassy yellow mineral from which sparks may readily be struck. The properties given here, however, appear to be a combination of those attributed to *heliotropium* and *topazos*. See also p. 46.

§ 22. Chalcedony is a form of silica. *Sineris* is *smyris*, or emery (an impure form

the stone which is called *Sineris*, and hanged about the neck, it is good against all fantastical illusions, and it maketh to overcome all causes, or matters in suit, and keepeth the body against thy adversaries.

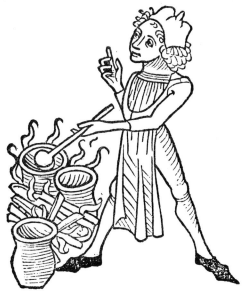

FIG. 14. *Hephaestites.*
From the *Hortus Sanitatis* (1491)

If thou wilt be acceptable,
and pleasant.

23

Take the stone which is called *Chelidonius*, and of it there is some black, and some somewhat red, and it is drawn out of

of corundum, Al_2O_3), and is the harder of the two stones, which explains its use here as an abrasive. 'Matters in suit', the translator's explanation of the Latin *causa*, refers in particular to law-suits.

§ 23. *Chelidonius*, the 'swallowstone' of Pliny, is a fabulous invention akin to the 'cockstone' (see *alectoria*, p. 32), and to other stones thought to be found in the bodies of animals (see *milvus*, p. 58). 'Old sicknesses and diseases' are illnesses that old people are susceptible to. The compiler of the Latin text has confused Albertus's *lunaticam passionem*, insanity, with *litargicam passionem*, a disease associated with lethargy; he also mis-transcribed Albertus's *epilepsiam*,

the belly of Swallows. If that which is somewhat red, be
wrapped in a linen cloth, or in a Calf's skin, and borne under
the left arm hole it is good against madness, and old sicknesses
and diseases, and the sleeping, or forgetful sickness, and
against *epidimia*, which is a scab that runneth through the whole
body. Evax saith that this stone maketh a man eloquent,
acceptable and pleasant. The black stone is good against wild
beasts, and wrath, and bringeth the business begun to an end.
And if it be wrapped in the leaves of Chelidonia, it is said
that it maketh the sight dull. And they should be drawn out
in the month of August, and two stones are found oftentimes
in one Swallow.

24   If thou wilt be victorious against
                        thy adversaries.

Take the stone which is called *Gagatronica*, and it is of divers
colours. The ancient Philosophers say that it hath been proved
in the prince Alcides, which how long he did bear it, he had
always victory. And it is a stone of divers colours, like the
skin of a Kid.

25   If thou wilt know before [of]
                        any thing to come.

Take the stone which is called *Hyaenia*, which is like a beast's
tooth, and put it under thy tongue. And as Aaron and the old

epilepsy, as *epidimiam*, the explanation of which the translator seems to have
invented. For a note on Evax, see Introduction, p. xxxv. *Chelidonia*, the celandine
or swallow-wort (*Chelidonium majus*), has been regarded since the time of
Dioscorides as having the power of improving the eyesight. The contradictory
statement here, Wyckoff points out, comes from Arnold (see Introduction,
p. xxxvi), and may be a confusion with *heliotropium*.

§ 24. The 'stone of Hercules' (Alcides was his patronymic) may possibly have
been amber (see *gagates*, p. 45), but the reference to 'divers colours' suggests
an iridescent stone, perhaps opal (a hydrated form of silica, SiO_2).

§ 25. *Hyaenia* stones, according to Pliny, are obtained from the eyes of the
hyena and may have been 'cat's eyes', quartz pebbles with a characteristic

Philosophers saith, how long thou wilt hold it so, always conjecturing, thou shalt prophesy things to come, and thou shalt not err in any wise for judging.

If thou wilt that thy garment be unable to be burned.

26

Take the stone which is called *Schistos*, which as Isidore saith, is like to saffron. And it is found in a part of Spain. This stone

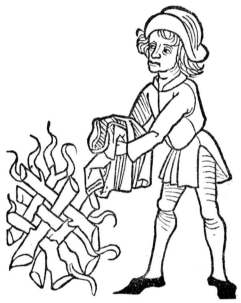

FIG. 15. *Schistos.*
From the *Hortus Sanitatis* (1491)

'chatoyant' sheen, due to included fine parallel needles of amphibole, $Ca(Mg,Fe)_2(SiO_2)_4$.

§ 26. *Schistos* is recorded by Albertus Magnus as *iscustos*. References to several different substances are included in this confused passage. Pliny says '*schistos* and haematite [iron oxide, Fe_2O_3] are closely related . . . Haematite is roasted, and bellows are used to fan it, until it turns red . . . *Schistos* has the same properties, in a weaker form . . . it is like saffron in colour' (xxxvi. 34. 144–5). The further properties stated here refer to asbestos (see p. 30); the sentence should read 'if this stone be made into a garment' (see illustration). Carbuncle bloweth like a pair of bellows, by reason of the windiness in it. It is found nigh the Gades of Hercules, that is two Isles, by the further parts of Spain beyond Granada, and if this stone be set in a garment it can be burned in no wise, but it shineth like fire. And some men say that the white Carbuncle stone is of this kind.

27
If thou wilt have favour
and honour.

Take the stone which is called *Kabrates*, and it is like to the Crystal stone. The ancient Philosophers, as Evax and Aaron, say of it that it giveth eloquence, favour and honour, and it is said moreover, that it healeth every dropsy.

28
If thou wilt drive away fantasies
and foolishness.

Take the stone which is called *Chrysolithus*, and it is of the same virtue with *Attemicus*, as Aaron and Evax say in the book of the natures of herbs, and stones. This stone, set in gold and borne, driveth away foolishness, and expelleth fantasies. It is affirmed to give wisdom, and it is good against fear.

is ruby (a red form of corundum, Al_2O_3); Pliny says some specimens 'cast a brilliant, colourless refulgence' and are called 'white carbuncles'. None of these minerals actually emits light. The compiler of the Latin text converted Albertus Magnus's *lapis filabilis propter viscositatem in eo arefactam*, 'a stone that splits into threads owing to the viscosity in it which has dried up' (Wyckoff), into *lapis flabilis est propter ventositatem in ipso rarefactam*, 'it is an airy stone owing to the windiness in it which is rarified'. The Gades of Hercules (*Gades Herculis* in the Latin text) are probably the Pillars of Hercules (*Columnae Herculis*), the mountains on either side of the Straits of Gibraltar. The straits were also known as *Gaditanum fretum*, 'the Straits of Gades', Gades being the modern Cadiz.

§ 27. *Kakabre* (p. 45) is the Arabic name for jet (*gagates*), but the stone intended here is a form of quartz (SiO_2).

§ 28. Chrysolite is a pale green form of olivine ($2(Mg, Fe)O.SiO_2$). In Pliny, it is a yellow transparent stone (topaz, $Al_2F_2SiO_4$); later, the names became transposed. *Attemicus* appears in some Latin texts as *aretico*; it appears to be a corruption of *arterica*, 'bronchitis' or 'asthma'.

If thou wilt judge the opinions   29
and thoughts of others.

Take the stone which is called *Gerachidem*, and it is of black colour. Let one hold it in his mouth, it maketh him that beareth it merry and in favour, and well esteemed with all men.

If thou wilt have victory   30
and amity.

Take the stone which is called *Nicomar*, and it is the same that is called Alabaster, and it is of a kind of Marble, and it is white and shining. And ointments are made of it for the bury⸗ ing of the dead.

If thou wilt that a man sleeping tell   31
to thee what he hath done.

Take the stone which is called *Quiritia*. This stone is found in the nest of the Lapwing or Black Plover.

If thou would obtain any   32
thing of any man.

Take the stone which is called *Radaim*, and it is black, shining through, which when the head of a Cock is given to Emmets

§ 29. Wyckoff makes the following correlations: Albertus Magnus, *gerachidem*; Damigeron (see p. xxxv), *gerachites*; Pliny, *hieracitis* (Greek, *hierax*, a falcon, referring to the dark grey colour); Albertus Magnus, *falcones*, which he says 'is called by another name, *arsenicum*'. Metallic arsenic is dark grey or black, but one should not take it into the mouth in search of euphoria.

§ 30. *Nicomar* is alabaster (a form of gypsum, $CaSO_4$). It is readily carved; here, references to its use in ancient times for ointment boxes and sarcophagi have been telescoped and misunderstood. Onyx marble (a form of calcite, $CaCO_3$) was used for the same purposes, and perhaps not clearly distinguished from alabaster.

§ 31. Lapwing, *Vanellus vanellus*. The Latin text, following Albertus Magnus, has hoopoe (*Upupa epops*), in this context. The ancient confusion between the two birds is mentioned in a note under *upupa*, p. 56.

§ 32. *Radaim* and *donatides* are alternative versions of the 'cockstone' (see

or Pismires to eat, it is found a long time after, in the head of
the Cock. And the same stone is also called *Donatides*.

33   If thou would make, that neither dogs, nor hunters
                 may hurt any beast, which they hunt.

Put before them the stone which is called *Liparea*, and they will
run soon to the stone. This stone is found in Libya, and all
beasts run to it, as to their defender. It letteth that neither dogs
nor hunters may hurt them.

34   If thou wilt burn any man's
                  hand without fire.

Take the stone which is called *Virites*, which we called before
Principen apii, which is fire, and it is as fire. If any man strain
hard this stone, it burneth soon his hand, like as it were burned
with a material fire, which is a marvellous thing.

alectoria, p. 32). A method of obtaining cleaned bones similar to that described
here is still used in natural history museums, where populations of the tiny
carrion-eating beetle *Dermestes lardarius* are used in preparing skeletons, in place
of 'emmets and pismires' (ants).

§ 33. Pliny says *liparea* was used for fumigation, and 'calls forth all beasts'.
Wyckoff suggests that it might have been sulphur from the Lipari Islands.
Marbod believes it to have a magic power of attracting wild animals; in
Albertus Magnus's version, where it is called *lippares*, it attracts and protects
them, though he has marked reservations about this. It is the latter account we
have here, shorn of Albertus's doubts. 'Letteth' here means 'preventeth'.

§ 34. *Virites* is pyrites (iron sulphide, FeS_2), and has been mentioned before,
under *peridonius*. The text is obscure: Albertus Magnus wrote *Virites est gemma
quam supra periritem diximus. Color autem ejus est fulgens ut ignis ut supra diximus*,
'Virites (pyrite) is the gem that we have called [*perithe*] above. Its colour is
brilliant like fire, as we have said before' (Wyckoff); the compiler of the Latin
text substituted the phrase *que prius diximus principē apii quod est ignis, et est ut ignis*,
of which we can make no more sense than the translator.

If thou wilt cure melancholy or   35
a fever quartan in any man.

Take the stone which is called *Lapis lazuli*. It is like to the colour of the heaven, and there is within it little bodies of gold. And it is sure and proved, that it cureth melancholy, and the fever quartan.

If thou would make any man's wit sharp and quick, and   36
augment his riches, and also prophesy things to come.

Take the stone which is called *Smaragdus*, in English speech an Emerald. And it is very clear, shining through and plain, but

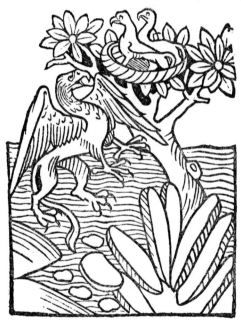

Fig. 16. *Smaragdus.*
From the *Hortus Sanitatis* (1491)

§ 35. Lapis lazuli (lazurite, $(Na,Ca)_8(S,Cl,SO_4)_4(AlSiO_4)_6$) frequently includes golden grains of pyrites ('fool's gold', FeS_2). The fever quartan is a fever which returns every third day.

§ 36. Emerald is now beryl ($3BeO.Al_2O_3.6SiO_2$), but in antiquity it was

it that is yellow is better. It is taken out of the nests of Grypes or Griffons. It doth both comfort and save, and being borne, it maketh a man to understand well, and giveth to him a good memory, augmenteth the riches of him that beareth it, and if any man shall hold it under his tongue, he shall prophesy anon.

37   If thou wilt make a rainbow
                                        to appear.

Take the stone which is called *Iris*, and it is white like to Crystal, four square or having horns. If this stone be put in the beam of the Sun, by turning back it maketh a rainbow soon to appear in the wall.

38   If thou wilt make a stone, which
                                   may never be made hot.

Take the stone which is called *Chalazia*. It hath the figure of hail and the colour and hardness of the Diamond. If this stone be put in a very great fire, it will never be hot. And the cause is, for it hath the holes so strait together, that the heat may not enter in the body of the stone. Also Aaron and Evax say, that

almost any green stone. The compiler of the Latin text seems to have mis-read Albertus's *viridissimus*, very green, as *mundissimus*, 'very clear' (Elyot). Pliny cites a 'yellow colour' as a flaw of *smaragdus*, and tells the griffin story about gold. Here 'griffin' is equated with 'grype' or vulture, *Gyps fulvus* (see p. 55).

§ 37. 'Iris' is Greek for 'rainbow'. What is referred to here is obviously a transparent crystal used as a prism. Albertus Magnus says iris stones are hexagonal, and thus must mean rock crystal (quartz, SiO_2). But the version here says 'four square', which suggests selenite (gypsum, $CaSO_4$); and 'having horns' is not a bad description of twinned crystals, a form in which selenite frequently occurs.

§ 38. *Chalazios* is Greek for 'hailstone', and what is intended here is probably a pebble of diamond or corundum; the fact that this would not be melted or damaged by fire has, Wyckoff suggests, been exaggerated to 'not even getting hot'. In the explanation which follows, heat is regarded as a fluid ('caloric'), and thought to enter bodies through invisible pores, in this case too contracted, 'strait', for any significant absorption. By sympathetic magic, the coldness of the stone is supposed to cool the 'heat' of anger or lust. See also *hyacinthus*, p. 47, and sapphire, p. 48.

this stone borne, mitigateth wrath, lechery and other hot passions.

If thou wilt know whether thy wife lieth with   39
any other married man, or no.

Take the stone called *Gagates* which is the same that is called *Kakabre*, and it is found in Libya and Britannia, the most noble Isle of the world, wherein is contained both countries, England and Scotland. It is of double colour; black, and of the colour of saffron, and it is found gray coloured, turning to paleness. It healeth the dropsy, and it bindeth the bellies that have a lax. And Avicenna saith, that if the stone be broken and washed, or be given to a woman to be washed, if she be not a virgin, she will piss soon, if she be a virgin, she will not piss.

If thou wilt overcome   40
thy enemies.

Take the stone which is called *Draconites*, from the Dragon's head. And if the stone be drawn out from him alive, it is good against all poisons, and he that beareth it on his left arm, shall overcome all his enemies.

If thou wilt engender love   41
between any two.

Take the stone which is called *Aetites*, and it is called of some *Aquileus*, because the Eagles put these in their nests. It is of

§ 39. *Gagates* is jet, a resinous, hard, coal-black variety of lignite ('brown coal'), capable of taking a high polish; *Kakabre* is the Arabic name for jet. The reference here to a yellow form ('the colour of saffron') is a confusion with amber; both of these semi-precious substances are found on seashores, are electrified by rubbing, and burn like incense—properties mentioned by Albertus Magnus, although not repeated here. The comment on Britain, inserted by the translator, is taken from Elyot's dictionary.

§ 40. *Draconites* is the 'snakestone', a fossil ammonite.

§ 41. *Aetites* or 'eaglestone' is Albertus Magnus's *echites*, and was a geode—a

purple colour, and it is found nigh the banks of the ocean sea, and sometimes in Persia, and it containeth always another stone in it, which soundeth in it when it is moved. It is said of ancient Philosophers that this stone, hanged up in the left shoulder, getteth love between the husband and his wife. It is profitable to women great with child; it letteth untimely birth; it mitigateth the peril of making afeared, and it is said to be good to them that hath the falling sickness. And as the men of Chaldea say, if poison be in thy meat, if the aforesaid stone be put in, it letteth that the meat may be swallowed down. And if it be taken out, the meat is soon swallowed down, and I did see that this last was examined sensibly of one of our brethren.

42   If thou wilt make a man sure.

Take the stone which is called *Hephaestites*. It is found in the sea; it is shining and ruddy. And it is said in the book of *Alchorath*, that if it be borne before the heart, it maketh a man sure, and refraineth and mitigateth all seditions, and discords. It is said also that it mitigateth the flies with long hinder legs which burneth corn with touching of it and devoureth the residue, fowls, clouds, hail, and such as have power of the fruits of the earth. And it hath been proved of Philosophers of late time, and of certain of our brethren, that it being put against the beam of the Sun putteth forth fiery beams. Also if this stone

hollow concretion containing crystals, a pebble, or earthy matter. Wyckoff points out that a stone which may be broken open to reveal another stone 'obviously suggested all the associated notions about eggs, fertility, pregnancy, etc.' The 'falling sickness' is epilepsy, and 'letteth' again means 'prevent(e)h'. 'The peril of making afeared' translates the Latin *perterritonis*, a misreading of Albertus Magnus's *parturitionis*, '[the dangers] of childbirth'.

§ 42. *Hephaestites*, recorded by Albertus Magnus as *epistrites*, is pyrites (iron sulphide, FeS_2). Part of this section has appeared before (see *hephaestites*, p. 36). Albertus Magnus says 'it is said to restrain locusts and birds and clouds and hailstorms, and to keep them off the crops' ('fruits of the earth'). The phrase 'the flies with long hinder legs . . .', etc., is Elyot's translation, or explanation, of the Latin word *locusta*. The 'book of *Alchorath*' has not been identified, though it may be a reference to Hippocrates (see Introduction, p. xli).

be put in seething water, the seething will soon cease, and the water will be cold a little after.

If thou wilt that strangers walk 43
sure and safe.

Take the stone which is called *Hyacinthus*, in English a Jacinth; it is of many colours. The green is best, and it hath red veins, and should be set in silver. And it is said in certain lectures that there is two kinds of it, of the water, and of the Sapphire. The Jacinth of the water is yellow white. The Jacinth of the Sapphire is very shining yellow, having no waterishness, and this is better. And it is written of this, in lectures of Philoso‐phers, that it being borne on the finger, or neck, maketh strangers sure, and acceptable to their guests. And it provoketh sleep for the coldness of it, and the Jacinth of Sapphire hath properly this [quality].

If thou wilt be saved from divers 44
chances and pestilent bites.

Take the stone which is called *Orites*, of which there be three kinds, one black, another green, and the third, of the which one part is rough and the other plain, and the colour of it is like the colour of plate of Iron; but the green hath white spots. This stone borne, preserveth from divers chances and perils of death.

§ 43. Albertus Magnus distinguishes two kinds of hyacinth; one is 'watery' (by which he apparently means 'transparent') and pale blue, and the other he calls *saphirinus* and says it is 'bright blue, having nothing watery about it; and this is more valuable'. The statement that 'the better kind is not quite transparent' he repeats elsewhere under *sappirus*. Albertus's word for 'blue', *blavus*, has been mistranscribed as *flavus* by the compiler of the Latin text, which accounts for the statement that the two kinds of stone are yellow. *Sappirus* for Pliny was lazuli, which is frequently veined, and though usually ultramarine in colour, may be a deep green, and perhaps this has been confused with *hyacinthus* here. 'Lectures' (Latin *lecturae*) are 'books'.

§ 44. Pliny says that *orites* (Greek, 'mountain stone') is the same as *sideritis* (Greek, 'iron stone'), which suggests that the third form at any rate might be magnetite (see *magnes*, p. 26).

45 If thou wilt make peace.

Take the stone which is called a Sapphire, which cometh from the East into India, and it that is of yellow colour is best, which is not very bright. It maketh peace and concord; it maketh the mind pure and devout toward God; it strengtheneth the mind in good things, and maketh a man to cool from inward heat.

46 If thou wilt cure vertigo.

Take the stone which is called *Samius*, from the isle Samos. It doth make firm or consolidate the mind of the bearer of it. And being bound to the hand of a woman travailing with child, it letteth the birth, and keepeth it in belly. Therefore it is forbidden in such a business that this stone touch a woman.

47 Thou shalt find many other like things in the Book of Minerals of Aaron and Evax.

48 The manner of doing these things consisteth in this, that the bearer, for a good effect, be clean from all pollution, or defiling of the body.

Explicit

49 Isidore seemeth to say that *Licania* hath in the head a stone of most noble virtue, and is of white colour; which, brayed,

§ 45. Albertus Magnus says: '*Sappirus* . . . comes from the East, from India. Its colour is . . . blue . . . and the better kind is not quite transparent.' See note under *hyacinthus*, p. 47.

§ 46. Terra Samia, along with other fine clays such as terra Lemnia and terra Cimolia (all named after their place of origin), had a long vogue as supposed antidotes to snake venom and other poisons. One variety, when dry, could be broken to show a star-like fracture, and was known as aster Samium; another variety, called collyrium, had a more leathery texture. A specimen of the latter is to be found in the pharmaceutical collection of Sir Hans Sloane (1660–1753) in the British Museum (Natural History).

§ 49. A confused passage. *Lyncurium* (Greek, 'lynx urine') was probably tourmaline (a complex fluoro-silicate) but was said by Theophrastus to be formed from the urine of the lynx, after the animal had buried it in sand. Isidore (see Introduction, p. xxxii) mentions *lyncurium* (xii. 2. 20 and xvi. 7. 8)

given to them that have the strangury to drink, it looseth perfectly the urine, and shortly healeth it, and putteth away the fever quartan. Also it taketh away a white spot or pearl in the eye. Also if a woman with child bear it on her she shall not lose her birth. Also the flesh of them sodden and eaten is good to them that have an exulceration, or sore in the lungs, with a consumption of all the body, and spitting of blood. Also the powder of the beasts, with the rind or bark of trees, with some grains of Pepper, is profitable against the haemorrhoids and growing out of flesh about the buttocks. Likewise they being raw, brayed with rinds or barks of trees, break ripe impostumes.

but does not credit it with the properties ascribed to it in the text. Here it is regarded as a 'headstone' (see *radaim*, p. 41), and reference is made to 'flesh', presumably of the lynx. The specimen from the medicine chest of Sir Hans Sloane is a belemnite (the internal shell of an extinct marine animal related to the cuttlefish). It has a radial internal structure, as is mentioned by Pomet in *A Compleat History of Drugges* (1712), where he says: 'At the End of the Stone there also appears, as it were, the Resemblance of a Sun.' 'Strangury' is obstruction of the urinary tract by organic concretions ('kidney stones'), and 'impostumes' are boils.

The Third Book of Albertus Magnus, of the Virtues of Certain Beasts

1 Forasmuch as it hath been spoken in the book before of certain effects caused by the virtue of certain stones, and of their marvellous virtue or operation, now we will speak in this chapter of certain effects caused of certain beasts.

Aquila	an Eagle
Tasso	[a Badger]
Bubo	a Shriek Owl
Hircus	a Goat Buck
Camelus	a Camel
Lepus	an Hare
Experiolus	[a Squirrel]
Leo	a Lion
Phoca	a Porpoise
Anguilla	an Eel
Mustela	a Weasel
Upupa	a Lapwing, or Black Plover
Pelicanus	a Pelican
Corvus	a Crow
Milvus	a Kite or Glede
Turtur	a Turtle [Dove]
Talpa	a Mole
Merula	a Black Mack or Ousel

2 *Aquila*, the Eagle, is a bird known enough. Of men of

§ 2. *Aquila chrysaëtos*, the golden eagle, is one of seven birds mentioned in this section proscribed as 'unclean' in Leviticus, but also held sacred in the ancient world. Hemlock (*Conium maculatum*) has been known from very early times to be an exceedingly poisonous herb. The symptoms are convulsions leading to paralysis without loss of consciousness, unless, as is usually the case, death supervenes. The explanation at the end of the paragraph is obscure; Aristotle

Chaldea it is called *Vorax*, and of the Greeks *Rimbicus*. Aaron and Evax say that it hath a marvellous nature or virtue; for if the brain of it be turned into powder, and be mixed with the juice of the Hemlock, they that eat of it shall take themselves by the hair, and they shall not leave the hold, so long as they

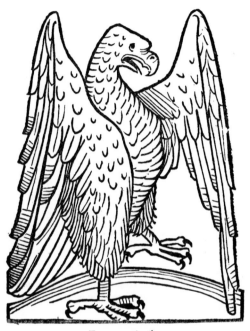

FIG. 17. *Aquila.*
From the *Hortus Sanitatis* (1491)

bear that they have received. The cause of this effect is for that the brain is very cold, insomuch that it engendreth a fantastical virtue, shutting the powers by smoke.

Tasso, [a Badger,] is a beast that is known well enough. It is ₃

thought of dry, smoky exhalations as potentially fiery, whilst the contrary cold exhalations were moist and clear. 'Fantastical' means 'of the mind, or imagination'.

§ 3. The feet and eyes of the badger (*Meles meles*) are said to confer invincibility, both by instilling fear, and by persuasion. The eyes of the lion and the 'lapwing' have a similar power.

called *Rapa* of the Chaldees, and of the Greeks *Orgalo*. Aaron saith of this, if the feet of it be borne of any man, he shall never be vexed, but he shall desire always to go forth. Also he that beareth the feet of it shall always overcome, and shall be feared of his enemies. And he said that his right eye, wrapped in a Wolf's skin, maketh a man pleasant, acceptable and gentle. And if meat be made of the aforesaid things, or powder given to any man in meat, the giver shall be greatly loved of him that receiveth it. This last was proved in our time.

4   *Bubo*, a Shriek Owl, is a bird well enough known; which is called *Magis* of the Chaldees, and *Hysopus* of the Greeks. There be marvellous virtues of this fowl, for if the heart and right foot of it be put upon a man sleeping, he shall say anon to thee whatsoever thou shalt ask of him. And this hath been proved of late time of our brethren. And if any man put this under his arm hole, no Dog will bark at him, but keep silence. And if these things aforesaid, joined together with a wing of it, be hanged up to a tree, birds will gather together to that tree.

5   *Hircus*, the Goat Buck, is a beast well enough known. It is called of the Chaldees *Erbichi*, of the Greeks *Massai*. If the

§ 4. *Tyto alba*, the barn owl, must be intended, for its call is a prolonged shriek; *Bubo bubo*, the eagle owl, makes brief guttural sounds. The two 'synonyms' here may originally have had some relevance to the text: the *magi* (see Introduction, p. xxxix) are translated elsewhere in this text as 'witches'; and *hysopus* is a Greek word of Hebrew origin, which always meant an aromatic herb (*Hyssopus officinalis*) used in temple purification ceremonies, so here perhaps it should be an additional ingredient in the recipe, and not a synonym. Owls generally are tabooed in Leviticus. The 'truth drug' effect of the heart of an owl is mentioned sceptically by Pliny: 'I will not omit a specimen of Magian fraud, for besides their other monstrous lies they declare that an horned owl's heart, placed on the left breast of a sleeping woman, makes her tell all her secrets' (xxix. 26. 81). Sympathetic magic (like attracting like) causing a 'miraculous assemblage', in this case of birds, recurs again under the porpoise and the mole.

§ 5. *Hircus* is classical Latin for he-goat. Fennel (*Foeniculum vulgare*) is an aromatic herb used mainly for culinary purposes. The blood of a goat was considered able to break a diamond (see p. 31), and so might be supposed to have at least some effect on glass. 'Sodden' means 'boiled'. Later we are told that the blood of the camel, as well as that of the goat, is hallucinogenic. The final sentence of the paragraph may have become displaced from the section on the eel, where it would appear to belong.

blood of it be taken warm with vinegar, and the juice of Fennel, and sodden together with a glass, it maketh the glass soft as dough, and it may be cast against a wall, and not be broken. And if the aforesaid confection be put in a vessel, and the face of any man be anointed with it, marvellous and

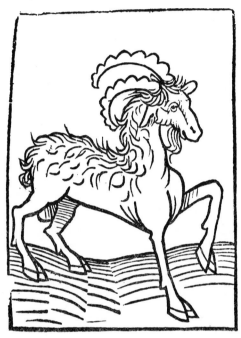

FIG. 18. *Hircus.*
From the *Hortus Sanitatis* (1491)

horrible things shall appear, and it shall seem to him that he must die. And if the aforesaid thing be put in the fire and there be there any man that hath the falling sickness, by putting to [him] the Loadstone, he falleth anon to the ground as dead, and if the water of Eels be given to him to drink, he shall be cured anon.

Camelus, the Camel, is a beast known well enough. It is 6

§ 6. *Stellio* is, literally, the spotted salamander (*Salamandra maculata*), but the passage may be an obscure alchemical cryptogram referring to some sort of

called of the Chaldees *Cyboi*, of the Greeks *Iphim*. If the blood of it be put into the skin of the beast called *Stellio*, which is like a lizard, having on his back spots like stars, and then set on any man's head, it shall seem that he is a giant, and that his head is in heaven. And this is said in the book of *Alchorath*, of Mercury. And if a lantern anointed with the blood of it be lightened, it shall seem that all men standing about have Camel's heads, so that there be no outward light of another candle.

7 *Lepus*, the Hare, is a beast well enough known. Of the Chaldees it is called *Veterellum*, and of the Greeks *Onollosa*. The virtue of it is shewed to be marvellous, for Evax and Aaron said that the feet of it, joined with a stone, or with the head of a Black Ousel, moveth a man to hardiness, so that he fear not death. And if it be bounden to his left arm, he may go whither he will and he shall return safe without peril. And if it be given to a Dog to eat, with the heart of a Weasel, from thenceforth he shall not cry out, although he should be killed.

8 *Experiolus*, [a Squirrel,] is a beast well enough known. If the claw of it be burned and consolidated, and be given in meat to any Horse, he will not eat for the space of three days. And if the aforesaid thing be put with a little Turpentine it shall be

distillation. The description of the salamander is taken from the Latin dictionary of Sir Thomas Elyot, who was apparently unable to identify the animal more precisely. 'Mercury' is Hermes Trismegistus, the first alchemist, cited as a source several times in the text. The magical 'perfuming' probably comes from the same source as the similar recipes in *The Marvels of the World*— see p. 97.

§ 7. *Lepus capensis*, the brown hare, an 'unclean' animal according to Leviticus, is here believed, like the badger, to confer invincibility. The silencing of the dog mentioned in the last sentence of the paragraph is to be attributed to the weasel's heart rather than to the hare's foot, for the statement is repeated under the weasel.

§ 8. The foot of the red squirrel (*Sciurus vulgaris*) is here said to be of use in bewitching horses; later we are told that the foot of the mole is even more efficacious. In the final sentence of the paragraph three stages in an alchemical experiment may be discerned—solution, precipitation, and a change in colour and consistency. With regard to the 'thunder', calcined bone, especially if still hot, when cast into a little water, might decrepitate.

clear, and secondly it shall be made as a cloud and blood, and if it be casten a little in water, an horrible thunder shall be made.

Leo, a Lion, is a beast well enough known, of the Chaldees 9 called *Balamus*, of the Greeks *Beruth*. If thongs of leather be made of the skin of him, and a man girded with them, he shall not fear his enemies. And if any man will eat of the flesh of him, and will drink of his water for three days, he shall be cured from the fever quartan. And if any part of his eyes be put under a man's arm hole and borne, all beasts shall flee away, bowing down their head unto their low bellies.

Phoca, a Porpoise, is a fish well enough known. Of the 10 Chaldees it is called *Daulaubur*, of the Grecians *Labor*. This fish is of diverse nature. If the tongue of it be taken, and be put with a little of the heart of it in water, for a surety fishes will gather there together. And if thou wilt bear it under thy arm hole, no man shall be able to have victory against thee; thou shalt have a gentle and pleasant judge.

Anguilla, an Eel, it is a fish sufficiently known. The virtues 11 of it are marvellous, as Evax and Aaron say, for if it die for fault of water, the heart remaining whole, and strong vinegar be taken, and it be mixed to the blood of the fowl called in Latin *Vultur*, which some call in English a Grype, and some

§ 9. The principle of sympathetic magic by association, which gives the lion (*Panthera leo*) the power to confer invincibility, is discussed at some length in the treatise at the beginning of the *Marvels of the World* (see pp. 74–6).

§ 10. *Phocaena communis*, the porpoise, rather than *Phoca vitulina*, the seal, is intended. Both animals, and also the eel, are taboo under Jewish law as 'fishes without scales'. The porpoise is of 'diverse nature' because it leaps from water to air, thus inhabiting two 'elements'. The recipe for causing a 'miraculous assemblage', in this case of fishes, is the second of three in this section (see under owl and mole), but this one would no doubt be more effective. The tongue and the heart of the porpoise are here considered to confer invincibility, whereas in other beasts it is the feet and eyes (see above, under *tasso*).

§ 11. *Anguilla anguilla*, the eel, was an 'unclean fish' (see under *phoca*). The griffin vulture (*Gyps fulvus*) is also tabooed in Leviticus. The sudden appearance in summer of large numbers of small black larval eels (elvers) in the estuaries of rivers gave credence to the idea that they were generated spontaneously from warm mud. There is a hint of this here, but present also is the notion that like is necessary to beget like. However, elvers are not poisonous.

a Raven, and be put under dung in any place, they shall all, how many soever they be, recover their life, as they had before. And if the worm of this Eel be drawn out, and put in the aforesaid confection the space of one month, the worm shall be changed into a very black Eel of which, if any man shall eat, he shall die.

12   *Mustela*, the Weasel, is a beast sufficiently known. If the heart of this beast be eaten yet quaking it maketh a man to know things to come, and if any Dog eat of the heart with the eyes and tongue of it, he shall soon lose his voice.

13   *Upupa*, the Lapwing or Black Plover, is a bird sufficiently known. Of the Chaldees it is called *Bori*, of the Greeks *Ison*. The eyes of it borne, make a man gross or great. And if the eyes of it be borne before a man's breast, all his enemies shall be pacified. And if thou shalt have the head of it in thy purse, thou canst not be deceived of any merchant. This hath been proved this day of our brethren.

14   *Pelicanus*, the Pelican, is a bird sufficiently known. It is called of the Chaldees *Voltri*, and of the Greeks *Iphalari*. The virtue of it is marvellous. If her young birds be killed and their heart not be broken, and if a part of her blood be taken and be put warm in the mouth of the young birds, they will

§ 12. *Mustela nivalis*, the weasel; in Greek, *cerdo*, a title applied to the goddess Demeter in her prophetic aspect. There may be some confusion between the mole and the weasel, for Pliny reports as a 'unique evidence of fraud' of the Magi their claim that the heart of the mole gives powers of divination (xxx. 6. 19). The 'tongue of it' mistranslates the Latin text, which has *lingua canis*, the herb hound's-tongue, said, on p. 9 above, to silence dogs.

§ 13. *Upupa epops* is the hoopoe; 'lapwing' (*Vanellus vanellus*) is a mistranslation of ancient origin. 'Lapwynge' for *Upupa* is given by Trevisa in his translation of Bartholemew's *De Proprietatibus Rerum* (1397), followed by Elyot's Latin Dictionary (1545). See also the illustration, p. 95. Here the bird is given as another example of an 'unclean' beast thought to confer invincibility.

§ 14. *Pelecanus onocrotalus*, the white pelican, is another tabooed bird. Following the tradition of Physiologus (see Introduction, p. xxxvii) the pelican was thought to be able to bring her young to life by feeding them with her own blood. The requirement that, for successful resuscitation, the hearts of the young birds must 'not be broken', is a touch of realism paralleled by a similar requirement in connection with the eels dead of drought (see p. 55).

receive soon again life as before. If it be hanged up to the neck of any bird, it shall fly always, until it fall dead. And the right foot of it under an hot thing, after three months shall be engendered quick, and shall move itself, of the humour and heat which the bird hath. And Hermes in the book of *Alchorath*, and Pliny doth witness this.

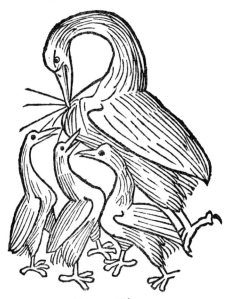

FIG. 19. *Pelecanus.*
From the *Hortus Sanitatis* (1491)

Corvus, called of some a Raven and of others a Crow. The 15 virtue of this fowl is marvellous, as Evax and Aaron rehearse. If her eggs be sodden, and be put again in the nest, the Raven

§ 15. Several birds of the family Corvidae appear to be confused here. *Corvus corone* is the common carrion crow. However, it is probably *Corvus corax*, the raven, a proscribed 'unclean' bird, which is intended, although the charming anecdote which follows about the bird taking stones of 'divers colours' into its nest would be more likely to apply to *Corvus monedula*, the jackdaw. 'Sodden' means 'boiled'. The magpie, similarly confronted with an attack on her nest, uses a herb to release bonds (see p. 99). 'After certain wise men' means 'according to certain wise men'. Of the stones mentioned above, *amandinus* (p. 32) fits the description best.

goeth soon to the Red Sea, in a certain Isle where *Aldoricus* or *Alodrius* is buried, and she bringeth a stone wherewith she toucheth her eggs, and the eggs be soon raw as they were before. It is a marvellous thing to stir up sodden eggs. If this stone be put in a ring, and the leaf of the Laurel tree put under it, and a man being bounden in chains, or a door shut, be touched therewith, he that is bounden shall soon be loosed, and the door shall be opened. And if this stone be put in a man's mouth it giveth to him understanding of all birds. The stone is of India, because it is found in India, after certain wise men, and sometimes in the Red Sea. It is of divers colours, and it maketh a man to forget all wrath, as we have said above in the same stone.

16   *Milvus*, a Kite or Glede, is a bird sufficiently known. Of the Chaldees it is called *Bysicus*, of the Greeks *Melos*. If the head of it be taken, and borne before a man's breast, it giveth to him love and favour of all men and women. If it be hanged to the neck of an Hen, she will never cease to run, until it be put away. And if a Cock's comb be anointed with the blood of it, he will not crow from thenceforth. There is a certain stone found in the knees of this bird, if it be looked craftily, which if it be put in the meat of two enemies, they shall be made friends, and there shall be made very good peace among them.

17   *Turtur*, a Turtle [Dove], is a bird well enough known. It is called *Mulon* of the Chaldees, of the Greeks *Pilax*. If the heart of this fowl be borne in a Wolf's skin, he that beareth it shall never have an appetite to commit lechery from thenceforth. If the heart of it be burned, and be put above the eggs of any fowl, there can never young birds be engendered of them from thenceforth. And if the feet of this fowl be hanged to a tree, it

§ 16. *Milvus milvus*, the kite, is tabooed in Leviticus. 'Stones' (calculi, bezoars) are sometimes though rarely found in the bladders of various animals, lending credence to the belief that they might be found elsewhere in the body. See the stones *alectoria* ('cockstone'), p. 32, and *chelidonius* ('swallowstone'), p. 37.

§ 17. *Streptopelia turtur*, the turtle dove, was the symbol of conjugal fidelity and passion, and the 'virtues' ascribed here, except possibly that against lechery, are out of place, belonging properly in the next paragraph under *talpa*.

shall not bear fruit from thenceforth. And if an hairy place, and an Horse, be anointed with the blood of it, and with water wherein that a Mole was sodden, the black hairs will fall off.

Talpa, a Mole, is a beast well enough known. The virtue of this beast is marvellous, as it is rehearsed of Philosophers. If 18

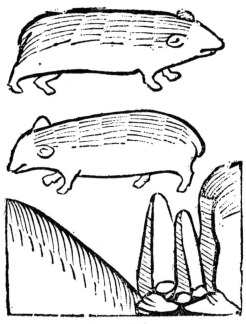

FIG. 20. *Talpa*.
From the *Hortus Sanitatis* (1491)

§ 18. The foot of the mole (*Talpa europaea*), in conjunction with the leaf of the laurel (see p. 4), is said here to be more effective than the foot of the squirrel (p. 54) in bewitching horses. Pliny says of the Magi that 'they look upon the mole of all living creatures with the greatest awe' (xxx. 6. 19). The *Hortus Sanitatis* (see Introduction, p. xliii) recommends the blood of a mole to make hairs grow rather than fall off (p. 71). Topsell (p. 391) explains the 'decoction' of the last sentence more fully: 'For the changing of hairs of Horses from black to white, take a Mole and boil her in salt water, or lye made of ashes, three days together . . . wash or bathe the place with the water or lye somewhat hot; presently the black hairs will fall . . . and in some short time there will come white.'

the foot of it be wrapped in the leaf of a Laurel tree, and be put in the mouth of an Horse, he will flee for fear. And if it be put in the nest of any fowl, there shall never come forth young birds of these eggs. And if thou wilt drive away Moles, put it in a pot, and quick Brimstone kindled, all the other Moles shall come together there. And the water of that decoction maketh a black Horse white.

19   *Merula*, a Black Mack or Ousel, is a fowl well enough known, and the virtue of it is marvellous. For if the feathers of the right wing of it, with a red leaf, be hanged up in the middle of an house which was never occupied, no man shall be able to sleep in that house, until it be put away. And if the heart of it be put under the head of a man sleeping, and he be inquired, he will say all that he hath done with an high voice.

20   The manner of doing all these beforesaid things, that the effect may be good and profitable, is that it be done under a favourable planet, as Jupiter and Venus, and this is in their days and hours. If any man therefore will do these things truly, without doubt he shall find truth, and very great effect or virtue, in the beforesaid things as I have proved, and seen oftentimes together with our brethren in our time. Therefore let him consider here, which shall find plenty of the beforesaid things, that he possesseth mastery and virtues. For if they be done in their contraries, as a good effect in a malicious sign, his virtue and effect should be letted for his contrary, and so good and true things should be despised. We see very many to be deceived, in sure and true things, which if they had

§ 19. *Turdus merula*, the blackbird, is no doubt intended here. The English translation of a work attributed to Michael Scott, *The Philosophers Banquet* (1614), includes the passages from *The Book of Secrets* on the owl, the mole, and the blackbird; the odd reference here to a 'red leaf' is probably the result of a misprint in the translator's Latin text (*folio* for *filo*), as Scott's version reads 'hung up . . . with a red thread'.

§ 20. This comment on the importance of astrology anticipates the section which follows (p. 62), in which the 'days and hours' of the planets, and their particular qualities, are explained. 'Letted' means 'prevented'.

known, and kept the qualities of signs, or times, they should have obtained their will and effect in the aforesaid things.

Isidorus seemeth to say, that the ashes of a great Frog, borne 21 at a woman's girdle, restraineth greatly the coming of a woman's natural purgation. And in a probation, if it be bounden to an Hen's neck, there shall come forth no blood of her, or of another beast. Also if it be tempered with water, and the head or another place be anointed with it, hair will no more grow there.

If any man bear a Dog's heart on his left side, all the Dogs 22 shall hold their peace, and not bark at him. If any man will bind the right eye of a Wolf on his right sleeve neither men nor Dogs may hurt him.

Here are ended some secrets of Albertus Magnus of Cologne upon natures, virtues, and effects of certain herbs, stones, and beasts. And here followeth in what hour every planet hath his dominion.

§ 21. The 'great frog' may be the edible species, *Rana esculenta*, distinguished by its slightly greater size and, from the time of Aristophanes, by its vocal exploits from the common frog, *R. temporaria*; but the toad (*Bufo bufo*), regarded as a magical creature from earliest times, may be intended. Isidore mentions none of the properties claimed here, but he does recommend, as a method of silencing dogs, a live frog given in meat (xii. 6. 58).

A Short Discourse of the Nature, and Qualities of the Seven Planets

1 And that all things which hath been said before, and also shall be said after, may be applied more easily to the effects of their desire which have not cunning of the stars, first thou shalt note that an hour is taken two ways, that is equal and unequal. The equal hour is the hour of the dial or clock, which is always equal. The unequal hour is considered, after that the days be longer or shorter. For the Astrologians consider always the time in the which the Sun standeth upon his half sphere and they call it the day, or the bow of the day, and by the contrary the night. They divide that time which they call the day in twelve equal parts, which be the hours of the same day, and whatsoever is said of the day, thou must understand contrari-wise of the night.

2 And that thou mayest understand more clearly, let us put the case, the Sun cometh out from his half sphere at four of the dial. We have unto the going down of the sun sixteen hours of the dial, which we may multiply by sixty as there be sixty minutes of every hour of the dial, and we shall have nine hundred and three score minutes, which we may divide by twelve as there be twelve hours of the day, applying to every hour his portion, and we have eighty minutes in an hour. Therefore every hour of the day shall have eighty minutes; which shall contain one hour and one third of an hour of the dial. And in all that time the dominion of the planet of that hour shall be considered, as the table beneath written shall show. Every hour of his night shall not have but forty minutes,

§§ 1–2. The astrological hours of the day are calculated by dividing into twelve equal parts the time between sunrise and sunset; naturally the length of these hours will change at different times of the year.

which thou shalt understand likewise of others, according to the rising of the Sun upon the ground; because that hour which is in the middle between night and day, which is called the dawning of the day, is not called the day, but the day is properly understood when the Sun may be seen.

Therefore [be] thou willing to consider the dominion of every 3 planet, for in every hour every planet hath his dominion; thou shalt consider the hours themselves, after the way above written, and so thou may come to the end of thy purpose. Also the beginning of the day is considered from one of the clock of the day, going before afternoon. So let the Sunday be divided into two equal parts, and it is of twelve hours, divide it into two, then the half day shall be eighteen and the first hour following shall be the beginning of Monday.

Wherefore, thou shalt consider that
4

> Sunday hath his sign under the Sun.
> Monday hath his sign under the Moon.
> Tuesday hath his sign under Mars.
> Wednesday hath his sign under Mercury.
> Thursday hath his sign under Jupiter.
> Friday hath his sign under Venus.
> Saturday hath his sign under Saturn.

It is to be noted that every true act must be done under his 5 planet. And it is better if it be done in the proper day of the planet, and in his own proper hour, as for an example:

under Saturn, life, building, doctrine, mutation;

§ 3. This last part is obscure. The beginning of the day astrologically is the hour starting at sunrise, which will vary with the time of year. The writer seems to suggest that we calculate the beginning of the day by counting eighteen ('unequal') hours from the previous noon, noon and midnight being the two hours which do not change with the season.

§ 5. Some years before the whole text of *The Book of Secrets* was translated, Thomas Moulton, in *The Myrour or Glasse of Helth* (1539), translated this section, at times more clearly. The influence of the sun, he said, gave 'esperance, gain, fortune and heritage', that of Venus 'love, society, loving and pilgrimage', and that of the moon 'sloth, evil thoughts and theft'. His translation of the Latin *palatium* as 'sloth' probably derives from reading it *paulatim*, 'gradually'.

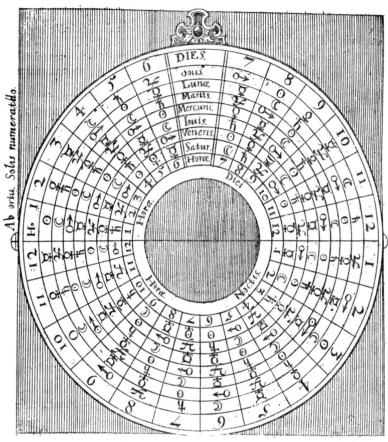

FIG. 21. Of the hours of the days and nights. The governing planet may be found
by reading the hours of the day (*horae diei*) counted from sunrise (*ab ortu solis*) and
finding the appropriate symbol in the circle for the day of the week: Sunday (*Solis*),
Monday (*Lunae*), Tuesday (*Martis*), Wednesday (*Mercurii*), Thursday (*Jovis*),
Friday (*Veneris*), or Saturday (*Saturni*). Each planet governs the first hour of its
day: the sun ⊙, the moon ☽, Mars ♂, Mercury ☿, Jupiter ♃, Venus ♀, and Saturn ♄.
The hours of the night (*horae noctis*) may be found in the same way. This diagram,
taken from Robert Fludd's *Utriusque Cosmi Historia* (Oppenheim, 1617), replaces
six pages of the original text which enumerate, less schematically, the same
information.

under Jupiter, honour, thing desired, riches, apparel;
under Mars, war, prison, matrimony, enemy;
under the Sun, hope, lucre, fortune, heir;
under Venus, friend or fellowship, way, lover, stranger;
under Mercury, loss, debt, fear;
under the Moon, palace, dream, merchandise, theft.

And note that Jupiter and Venus be good, Saturn and Mars 6
evil, but the Sun and the Moon in a mean; and Mercury is
good with good and evil with evil.

S A T U R N is the highest planet, whose nature is cold and dry, 7

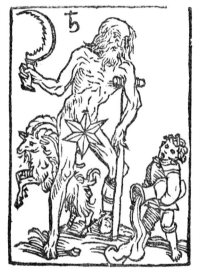

FIG. 22. Saturn.
From *Naturalia Alberti Magni* (1548)

§ 7. Added in the later Elizabethan editions, these descriptions of the nature of
the seven planets go into far more detail than the original Latin. The edition
of 1599 had small illustrations of the seven planets; the illustrations used here,
like those of the herbs, were taken from the German edition of 1548. Saturn
was equated by the Romans with Cronos, in Greek mythology the king of the
gods before Zeus; Cronos in turn became associated with Chronos (Time) and
was said to govern old age—hence he is shown in the illustration with a sickle
and a crutch. The two 'houses' or signs of the zodiac connected with Saturn

whose complexion melancholic, an enemy to mankind, masculine, of the day, evil disposed, and counted the greater misfortune. He is of slow motion, for he performeth his course but in thirty years. He governeth in a man's body the right ear, the milt, the bladder. He hath dominion over the phthisic, catarrh, palsy, dropsy, quartan ague, consumption, gout, leprosy, morphew, cancer, flux, and griefs of the spleen. He is a friend to the retentive faculty, and he hath two houses as *Capricorn* and *Aquarius*. If he be Lord of the nativity, he maketh the children of proud heart, lofty in honours, sad, keeping anger, upright in counsel, disagreeing with their wives, malicious; of stature lean, pale, slender, and hard favoured, thick lips, wide nostrils and cold of nature. This planet giveth denomination to Saturday, because he ruleth the first hour of the day.

8 JUPITER is next beneath Saturn, whose nature is warm and moist, whose complexion sanguine, a friend to nature and to mankind, masculine, of the day, and called the greater fortune; he is meetly slow of motion, performing his circuit but in twelve years. He governeth in a man's body the liver, the

are Capricorn, the goat, which represents the masculine aspect, and Aquarius, the water-carrier, representing the feminine. Saturn's qualities, cold and dry, associate it also with the element earth and the melancholic 'humour' or 'complexion' which had its origin in the spleen (the 'milt'). Phthisic is tuber-culosis, the quartan ague a malarial fever which returns every third day, mor-phew a disease of the skin, and the flux a fluid discharge, usually diarrhoea.

§ 8. Jupiter, or Jove, corresponding to the Greek Zeus, was lord of the heavens; hence his baton and arrows (thunderbolts) in the illustration. Sagit-tarius, the archer, is the masculine manifestation of Jupiter, Pisces, the fish, the feminine. His humour is jovial, or sanguine, warm and moist, associated with the blood and the element air. Of the importance of blood, Sir Thomas Elyot in *The Castel of Helth* (1534) writes 'Blood hath pre-eminence over all other humours in sustaining of all living creatures, for it hath more conformity with the original cause of living, by reason of temperance in heat and moisture . . . The distemperance of blood happeneth by one of the other three humours, by the inordinate or superfluous mixture of them' (fol. 8). The ideal state of man was a balance between the four qualities and humours, and the sanguine comes closest to such even temper. The 'king's evil' is scrofula, a disease of the throat causing swollen glands.

lungs, the ribs, midriff, gristles, blood and seed. He hath dominion over the King's evil, pleurisy, infection of the lungs, apoplexy proceeding of blood, cramp, great headache, heart-burning, and other diseases rising of blood. He helpeth the digestive and nutritive faculties, and he hath likewise two

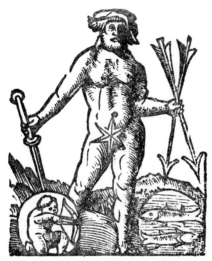

FIG. 23. Jupiter.
From *Naturalia Alberti Magni* (1548)

houses, *Sagittarius* and *Pisces*. If he be Lord of the nativity, he maketh the children born to be of notable courage, trusty, achieving great exploits, merry, glorious, honest; of stature fair and lovely coloured, gentle eyes, thick hair, stately in going, very loving both of wife and children. He giveth name to Thursday, because he ruleth the first hour of that day.

MARS followeth Jupiter, whose nature is immoderate hot and 9

§ 9. Mars, god of war, is illustrated with helmet, sword, and battle-axe; his association with the element fire is shown by the flaming brand. Aries, the ram, represents the masculine aspect of Mars, and Scorpio, the scorpion, the feminine. War and anger are the result of the choleric humour, which, according to Elyot, is 'the foam of blood, the colour whereof is red and clear, or more like to orange colour, and is hot and dry, wherein the fire hath dominion . . . whose beginning is the liver' (fol. 9). Since astrology originally recognized seven

dry, whose complexion choleric, masculine, of the night, evil disposed, and termed the lesser misfortune. He is indifferent quick of motion, performing his course in two years. He governeth in a man's body the left ear, the gall, the reins, and cods. He hath influence in the tertian fever, pestilence, and

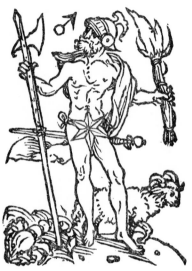

FIG. 24. Mars.
From *Naturalia Alberti Magni* (1548)

continual ague, ringworm, megrim, rottenness, untimely deliverance, breaking of veins, and all diseases caused by choler, and hath two mansions, *Aries* and *Scorpio*. If he be Lord of the nativity, he maketh the children born rough, wild, fierce, invincible, bold, contentious, obscure, easy to be deceived; of stature indifferent, lean, hard faced, red headed, small eyed, delighting to burn and destroy, subject to breaking their limbs, and violent death, or else to fall down from an

'planets' (the sun, the moon, and the five planets then known), while there are only four Aristotelian elements, some sharing of properties is necessary, so the 'hot and dry' of Mars is distinguished from the corresponding attributes of the sun as 'immoderate'. Megrim is migraine, the 'tertian' a malarial fever that returns every other day; the reins are the kidneys and the cods the testicles.

high place. This planet giveth denomination to Tuesday, because he ruleth the first hour of that day.

SOL, or the Sun, ensueth next Mars, whose nature is hot and 10 dry moderately, the life and light of all the other planets; masculine, of the day, good fortune by aspect, but evil fortune

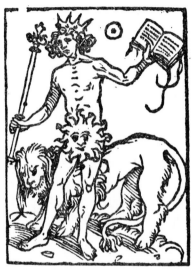

FIG. 25. The Sun.
From *Naturalia Alberti Magni* (1548)

by corporal conjunction. He is quick of motion, finishing his course in three hundred forty five days, and almost six hours. He governeth in man's body the brain, marrow, sinews, the right eye of a man and the left eye of a woman. He hath rule

§ 10. The astrological supremacy of the sun is symbolized by a sceptre, and the sun's association with Apollo, god of prophecy and poetry, is shown by the book. Though hot and dry, the sun is not choleric, as is Mars; rather he represents the essence of the masculine qualities—as the conveniently placed sun in the illustration suggests. Like the moon, which correspondingly represents the feminine, the sun has only one sign, Leo, the lion. The times of motion for the outer planets are remarkably accurate, if we accept that a misreading has occurred here; to the nearest hour, the duration of the solar year is 365 days and 6 hours. In Roman numerals the number CCCLXV could easily be transposed to become CCCXLV.

of all hurts in the mouth, in distillations from the eyes, and in all hot and dry diseases which proceed not of choler, and hath but only one mansion; to wit, *Leo*. If he be Lord of the nativity he maketh the children born trusty, lofty, wise, just, courteous, religious, and obedient unto their parents; of person corpulent, their hair inclined to yellow, tall, large limbed, doing all things with a grace; and if this planet be well placed, he causeth long life. This planet giveth denomination to Sunday, because he ruleth the first hour of that day.

11 VENUS runneth after *Sol*, whose nature is cold and moist

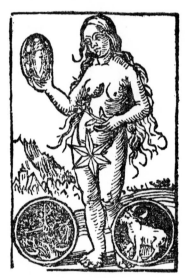

FIG. 26. Venus.
From *Naturalia Alberti Magni* (1548)

§ 11. In the illustration, Venus is carrying her traditional symbol, a hand mirror, and a herb which might be *Legousia hybrida*, called 'Venus looking-glass' by Gerard. Libra, the scales, signifies the masculine side of Venus, and Taurus, the bull, rather oddly represents the feminine. Venus, or Aphrodite, goddes of love, was born from the foam of the sea, and is associated with the elemen, water and the phlegmatic humour. In the Ptolemaic model of the universe, with the Earth in the centre, the inner planets (Venus and Mercury) were thought to revolve around the earth in the same period as the sun; the movements of the planets independent of the sun were explained by the planets'

temperately: whose complexion phlegmatic, feminine, of the night, and is cleped the lesser fortune, but of inclination well disposed to mankind. She is of a swift progression, absolving her revolution in one year. She governeth in man's body the loins, kidneys, buttocks, belly, flank and matrix. She beareth rule over all cold maladies, and moist, in the liver, heart, and stomach, and specially women about their privities; and she hath two mansions or houses, *Taurus* and *Libra*. If she be Lady of the nativity, she maketh the children born pleasant, merry, given to pleasures, lovely, lecherous, just, inviolable keepers of faith and friendliness; of stature tall, comely, white and fair, having wanton and amiable eyes, gentle looks, thick and soft hair, sometimes curled, dancers and delighted in music. This gentle planet giveth denomination to Friday, because she ruleth the first hour in that day.

MERCURY immediately followeth Venus, whose nature in all 12 respects is common and convertible: masculine with masculine, feminine with feminine, hot with hot, cold [with cold], moist with moist, dry with dry, good fortune with good fortune, best with a good aspect or conjunction. He is of swift motion, going his course in a year. He governeth in man's body the tongue, memory, cogitation, hands and thighs. He hath dominion over the frenzy, madness, melancholy, falling sick⁄ ness, cough, rheum and the abundance of distilling spittle, and generally all things are subject unto him; and he hath two

additional movement on an 'epicycle', a moving circle on the surface of the sphere. Venus in fact completes her orbit around the sun in 226 days. 'Cleped' means 'called'; the matrix is the womb.

§ 12. Mercury was equated by the Romans with the Greek Hermes, who carried a caduceus, or staff with two snakes entwined round it; in the illustration the snakes are evident, but the staff itself has disappeared. Hermes was also god of wealth, so he is shown clutching a moneybag. The sign Gemini, the twins, represents the masculine in Mercury, Virgo, the virgin, the feminine. The problem of associating seven planets with only four basic elements was overcome by assigning all possible combinations of qualities to Mercury; hence a person with a mercurial temper is likely to be changeable in humour. The orbit of Mercury is completed in 88 days (see the note to Venus). 'Stout' means 'brave'.

mansions, *Gemini* and *Virgo*. If he be Lord of the nativity, he maketh the children stout, wise and apt to learn, modest, secret, and eloquent; of person small, lean, pale of visage, smooth haired, fair eyed, hard and bony handed. This planet

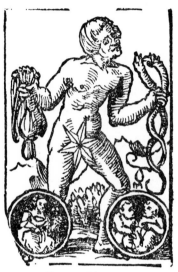

Fig. 27. Mercury.
From *Naturalia Alberti Magni* (1548)

giveth name to Wednesday, because he ruleth the first hour in that day.

13 LUNA, or the Moon, cometh last, and lowest of all the planets; whose nature is cold and moist, feminine and of the night, conveyor of the virtue of all other planets coming next from her to us. She is of a very passing swift motion, finishing her course in twenty-seven days, seven hours, and forty-four minutes. She governeth in a man's body the brain, the left eye

§ 13. The moon is illustrated in the form of the goddess Diana, or Artemis, with hunting horn and spear. The lobster is a curious variation of Cancer, the crab, the 'house' assigned to the moon. Complementary to the sun, the moon is the essence of the feminine, cold and moist like Venus, and, of course, changeable. 'Writhing of the body' and 'displaying of members', references to fits and diseases of nervous origin, are related to the moon's power over lunacy.

of a man and the right eye of a woman, the privy parts of a woman, the stomach both in man and woman, the belly, and generally all the left parts of the body. She ruleth the palsy and writhing of the body, displaying of members, obstruction of sinews, with infirmities proceeding of cold moisture, and she

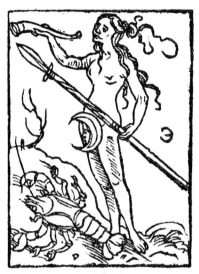

FIG. 28. The Moon.
From *Naturalia Alberti Magni* (1548)

hath but one house only, to wit, *Cancer*. If she be Sovereign of the nativity, she maketh the children born honest, honourable, inconstant, loving wet and moist places, and given to see strange countries; of stature tall, white and effeminate. She giveth name to Monday, because she ruleth the first hour in that day.

Here beginneth the Book of the Marvels of the World, set forth by Albertus Magnus

1 After, it was known of Philosophers that all kinds of things move and incline to themselves, because an active and ration‑able virtue is in them, which they guide and move, as well to themselves as to others, as fire moveth to fire, and water to water.

2 Also Avicenna said, when a thing standeth long in salt, it is salt, and if any thing stand in a stinking place, it is made stinking. And if any thing standeth with a bold man, it is made bold; if it stand with a fearful man, it is made fearful. And if a beast companieth with men it is made tractable and familiar. And generally it is verified of them by reasons, and diverse experience, that every nature moveth to his kind, and their verifying is known in the first qualities, and likewise in the second and the same chanceth in the third. And in all dispositions there is nothing which moveth not to itself, accord‑ing to his whole power. And this was the root, and the second

The translator has omitted, perhaps censored, a long introductory passage dealing with the effects of sorcery. The Latin writer, assuming that all men admit the efficacy of magic, sets out to explain how it works. He does this by quoting Avicenna and the authors of books on necromancy to the effect that the soul of man can alter material objects, under the right conditions. He then sets out to establish the general principles by which 'marvels' may be understood.

§ 1. The first principle is affinity, attraction between things with similar qualities or virtues, here stated in general terms, referring to the Aristotelian elements—earth, air, fire, and water. The meaning of 'rationable' is obscure; it may have the sense 'moderate', 'discriminating' or (related to mathematical 'ratio') it may mean 'proportionable' or 'variable'.

§ 2. The second principle: all things have prime (or first) qualities, but can acquire second (and maybe third) qualities by association, to which the principle of affinity applies also. Throughout this section the translator has used 'experience' for what we would understand as 'experiment'.

beginning of the works of secrets. And turn thou not away the eyes of thy mind.

After that, this was grafted in the minds of the Philosophers 3 and they found the disposition of natural things. For they knew surely that great cold is grafted in some, in some great boldness, in some great wrath, in some great fear, in some barrenness is engendered, in some ferventness of love is engendered, in some is some other virtue engendered; either after the whole kind, as boldness and victory is natural to a Lion, or *secundum individuum*, as boldness is in an harlot, not by Man's kind, but *per individuum*. There came of this great marvels and secrets able to be wrought. And they that understood not the marvellousness, and how that might be, did despise and cast away all things in which the labour and wit of Philosophers was, whose intent and labour was their own praise in their posterity, that they might by their writing make things called false, in great estimation.

It is not secret and hidden to the people, that every like 4 helpeth and strengtheneth his like, and loveth, moveth and embraceth it. And Physicians have now said and verified that for their part, and have said that the liver helpeth to the liver, and every member helpeth his like. And the turners of one metal into another called Alchemists know that by manifest truth, how like nature secretly entereth, and rejoiceth of his like. And every science hath now verified that in his like. And note thou this diligently, for great marvellous works shall be seen upon this.

Now it is verified and put in all men's minds, that every 5

§ 3. The third principle: qualities may be innate to a whole species ('whole kind'), or to individual things; they were called by Aristotle 'essential' and 'accidental' qualities respectively. 'Engendered' is a literal translation of *innatus*, 'innate'; 'grafted' is used in the sense 'instilled', here and elsewhere.

§ 4. Here the principle of affinity is reasserted, this time referring to more specific objects than the basic elements.

§ 5. The fourth principle, antagonism: as all things 'attract' things with like qualities, so they 'repel' things with opposite qualities. The third principle (qualities innate to a whole species or an individual) applies to antagonism as well as to affinity. Timbrels, tabors, and drumslades are different kinds of drums.

natural kind, and that every particular or general nature, hath natural amity and enmity to some other. And every kind hath some horrible enemy, and destroying thing to be feared; likewise something rejoicing exceedingly, making glad, and agreeing by nature. As the Sheep doth fear the Wolf, and it knoweth not only him alive, but also dead; not only by sight, but also by taste; and the Hare feareth the Dog and the Mouse the Cat, and all four-footed beasts fear the Lion, and all flying birds flee the Eagle and all beasts fear Man, and this is grafted to every one by nature. And some have this *secundum totam speciem*, and at all times, but some only *secundum individuum*, and at a certain time. And it is the certifying of all Philosophers, that they which hate other in their life, hate their parts altogether after they die. For a skin of a Sheep is consumed of the skin of the Wolf; and a timbrel, tabor or drumslade made of the skin of a Wolf causeth [that] which is made of a Sheep's skin not to be heard, and so is it in all others. And note thou this for a great secret.

6   And it is manifest to all men that Man is the end of natural things, and that all natural things are by him, and he overcometh all things. And natural things have natural obedience grafted in them to Man, and Man is full of all marvellousness, so that in him are all conditions; that is mistemperance in heat and cold, [but] temperate in every thing that he will. And in him be the virtues of all things, and all secret arts worketh in man's body itself, and every marvellous thing cometh forth of him; but a man hath not all these things at one time but in divers times, and in *diversis individuis*. And in him is found the effect of all things. Thou shalt note how much reason may see and comprehend, and how much thou may prove by experience, and so understand that which is against Man.

§ 6. The fifth principle, anthropocentricity: the 'final cause' in Aristotle's sense of 'purpose' of all things is Man. But here, coupled with this typically medieval view, is the modern-sounding idea that Man can overcome his imperfections ('temperate in everything that he will') and that his potentialities are limitless when different individuals co-operate over a period of time.

There is no man but doth know that every thing is full of 7 marvellous operations, and thou knowest not which is [of] greatest operation, till thou hast proved it. But every man despiseth the thing whereof he knoweth nothing, and that hath done no pleasure to him. And every thing hath of hot and cold, that is proper to him, and fire is not more marvellous than water, but they are diverse and after another manner; and Pepper is not more marvellous than Henbane, but after another fashion. And he that believeth that marvellousness of things cometh from hot and cold, can not but say that there is a thing to be marvelled in everything, seeing that every thing hath of heat and cold that is convenient to it.

And he that believeth that marvellousness of things be in 8 stars (of which all things take their marvellous and hidden properties) may know that every thing hath his proper figure celestial agreeing to them, of which also cometh marvellousness in working. For every thing which beginneth, beginneth under a determinate ascendant and celestial influence, and getteth a proper effect, or virtue of suffering, or working a marvellous thing. And [there is] he that believeth that the marvellousness of things cometh by amity and enmity, as buying and selling can not be denied so for to come. And thus universally every thing is full of marvellous things, after every way of searching the natures of them. And after that the Philosophers knew this, they began to prove and say what is in things.

§ 7. After a statement that all properties must be tested by experiment or proof, the sixth principle is established: the natures of all things are determined by the proportions of the Aristotelian qualities hot and cold (the 'active' qualities), dry and moist (passive), which in different combinations give rise to the four elements. Pepper is hot and dry, henbane (see p. 10), according to Turner, is 'cold in the third degree'.

§ 8. The seventh principle, astrology: the qualities, active and passive ('effect or 'suffering'), of all things are determined by the 'celestial figure' (i.e. the positions of the planets with reference to the 'fixed' stars) at the time of their beginning. The reference to the fourth principle (antagonism) might more properly belong to the next paragraph, where those things necessary for a complete knowledge of 'marvellousness' are listed.

9   Plato saith in *Libri Regimenti* that he that is not an expert in Logic, of which the understanding is made ready, lifted up, nimble or light and speedy; and he that is [not] cunning in Natural Science, in which are declared marvellous things, both hot and cold, and in which the properties of every thing in itself be showed; and [he] which is not cunning in the science of Astrology and in the aspects and figures of stars, of which every one of them which be high hath a virtue and property; can not understand nor verify all things which Philosophers have written, nor can certify all things which shall appear to Man's senses, and he shall go with heaviness of mind, for in those things is marvellousness of all things which are seen.

10   A pure Astrologian believeth that all marvellousness of things, and that the root of experience, and of all things which be apparent when they be put together, were from a celestial figure which every thing getteth in the hour of his killing or generation. And he hath verified it; in every thing that he hath proved he findeth that the concourse of things is according to the course of the stars. And victory, joy and heaviness, dependeth thereof, and is judged by it. And therefore he commanded all things to be done in certain days, in certain hours, in certain conjunctions, and separations, in certain ascensions. And their wit could not attain to all the knowledge of Philosophers.

11   A great part of Philosophers and Physicians hath believed

§ 9. The pseudo-Plato's authority (see Introduction, p. xlii) is invoked to support a reassertion of the necessity for (i) a knowledge of and the ability to apply the principles enumerated above ('Logic'); (ii) a knowledge of Aristotelian qualities ('Natural Science'); and (iii) astrology. Again a reference to magic has been omitted; the Latin text includes (iv) a knowledge of necromancy.

§ 10. Astrology, though a complex and highly developed art, is not able to explain everything; the 'pure Astrologian' sees only a part of the sum total of knowledge. The phrase 'all things which be apparent when they be put together' might better have been translated 'all things which are proved [by the facts] when they be compared'.

§ 11. Similarly those who try to explain everything in the terms of natural science discover that they see only a part of the truth, evidenced by their inability to fit observed experience to theory.

that all that marvellousness of experience and marvels came from natural things, when they be brought to light, by hot and cold, dry and moist; and they showed these four qualities, and put them to be the roots of all marvellous things, and the mixtion of them is required for every marvellous thing. They verified that in their works. And when they found [by] many experiences of Philosophers [that] they might not verify those things by hot and cold but rather by his contrary, it chanceth them to marvel continually, and to be sorry, and to deny that oftentimes, although they see it.

Therefore Plato said for a good cause, that he which is not 12 very cunning in Logic, and wise in the virtues of natural things, likewise the aspects of the stars, shall not see the causes of marvellous things, nor know them, nor participate of the treasure of Philosophers.

Therefore I know that every thing hath that which is his 13 own of heat and cold (of which it maketh another thing effectual by accident, directly and indirectly) and it hath all his virtues of the stars, and the figure of his generation, which worketh in mortality, construction, and agreeing with others. And notwithstanding, every thing hath his own natural virtues, by which every thing is a beginning of a marvellous effect. Therefore seeing that every nature moveth to his own like, it may be imagined of the marvellousness of effects, to work every thing that thou wilt. And thou shalt verify it in all things which thou shalt hear, both of Physic and all other Natural Sciences, after a diverse way of thy thought and wit. And I shall show thee manifestly, that thou mayest help thy self, and prepare thee to receive those things which I will tell to thee,

§ 12. The author's contention, following the authority of 'Plato', that all kinds of knowledge are necessary for full understanding is repeated, following his demonstration that the specialist cannot explain all phenomena.

§ 13. Armed with knowledge of all these subjects, the reader may 'help himself', an exhortation to individual thought which adds a modern note to the discussion. 'By accident' refers again to Aristotle's 'accidental' qualities (see note, p. 75); 'a beginning of a marvellous effect' means 'the origin of a marvellous effect'.

gathered and collected of Philosophers and divers ancient authors.

14   Therefore have thou this thing in thy mind, that an hot thing, as much as it is by itself, helpeth in cold passions (and it is proved in them) and agreeth not to hot things, but by accident or indirectly. That which is by accident, may deceive thee in the first qualities, for oftentimes an hot thing healeth hot sicknesses, that is by accident or indirectly. Therefore, if thou wilt have experience: first it becometh thee to know of things whether they be hot or cold, and note all that. And after thou knowest that, note what is the disposition and natural properties of it, whether is it boldness or fearfulness, or honesty, or barren-ness; for of what nature every thing hath, he is like to such in these things in which he is associate. As the Lion is a beast unfearful, and hath a natural boldness, chiefly in his forehead and heart. And therefore he that taketh in his fellowship the eye or heart of a Lion, or the skin which is between his two eyes, goeth bold and not fearful, and bringeth fearfulness to all beasts. And generally there is in a Lion virtue to give boldness and magnanimity. Likewise in an harlot boldness is extreme. And therefore Philosophers say if any man put on a common harlot's smock, or look in the glass (or have it with him) in which she beholdeth herself, he goeth bold and unfearful. Likewise there is great boldness in a Cock, in so much that Philosophers say that the Lion is astonished when he seeth him. And therefore they say, if any man bear any thing of his, he goeth boldly.

15   And generally every beast which hath boldness extreme by

§ 14. After a statement of the Aristotelian view that reactions take place through contrary qualities, the principle of affinity is re-stated in order to give examples of the way marvels may be accomplished by sympathetic magic. The English translator, following the Latin, has 'exterminate' for 'extreme' (l. 20), a corruption which contradicts the sense of the passage. The story about the lion being afraid of a white cock is told by Pliny (x. 24. 47).

§ 15. The sentence (conjecturally reconstructed) which leaves the Latin un-translated, may be rendered: 'If anything of this sort were fashioned from it, it giveth to him [the possessor] boldness.' In the example which follows, premature birth is, curiously, linked with castration. The 'stones' are the testicles, the

nature or chance, *si [quid] ex eo construeretur huiusmodi*, it giveth to him boldness. Likewise if it be a barren beast, by nature or by some accident followed to it, it moveth some to barrenness. And therefore Philosophers have written that the Mule, forasmuch as he is utterly barren of his property, and whosoever it be, maketh men and women barren, when some part of him is associate to women. And likewise doth he that was born afore the natural time, and a gelded man, because barrenness is grafted in all these. And they make like themselves in this a man which doth associate to himself these inward things. Likewise they which will move love look what beast loveth most greatly, and specially in that hour in which it is most stirred up in love, because there is then greater strength in it in moving to love; they take a part of the beast, in which carnal appetite is stronger, as are the heart, the stones, and the mother or matrix.

And because the Swallow loveth greatly, as Philosophers 16 saith, therefore they choose her greatly to stir up love.

Likewise the Dove and the Sparrow are holden to be of this 17 kind, specially when they are delighted in love, or carnal appetite, for then they provoke and bring in love without resistance.

Likewise when they will make a man to be a babbler, or of 18 much speech, they put nigh to him a part of a Dog's tongue or heart, but when they will make a man eloquent or delightable, they associate to him a Nightingale; and to speak universally, whatsoever virtue or natural property they see in any natural thing after an excess, they thought to make like to move or incline any thing disposed to that same. For they know surely that it might more help than hurt, in so much as it hath grafted in it of their nature. And all virtue moveth to such as it is, according to the power of it. And so must thou understand it to be in marvellous things, of which thou shalt hear. And this is said to introduce thy mind.

'mother or matrix' the womb. Further examples of sympathetic magic are given in the next three paragraphs.

19   The author [of] *Libri Regimenti* saith that there be certain things manifest to the senses in which we know no reason. And certain be manifest by reason, in which we perceive *nullum sensum nec sensationem*. And in the first kind of things we must believe no man, but experience; and reason is to be proved by experience not to be denied. And in the second kind of things feeling is not to be looked for, because it may not be felt. Therefore certain things must be believed by only experience, without reason, for they be hid from men; certain [things] are to be believed by only reason, because they lack senses.

20   For although we know not a manifest reason wherefore the Loadstone draweth to it Iron, notwithstanding experience doth manifest it so, that no man may deny it. And like as this is marvellous, which only experience doth certify, so should a man suppose in other things. And he should not deny any marvellous thing although he hath no reason, but he ought to prove by experience; for the cause of marvellous things are hid, and of so diverse causes going before, that man's understanding, after Plato, may not apprehend them. Therefore the Loadstone draweth Iron to it, and a certain other stone draweth glass. So marvellous things are declared of Philoso-

§ 19. The eighth principle combines a medieval view with an almost scientific attitude. The Latin '*nullum sensum nec sensationem*' is obscure; the larger passage is freely translated by Thorndike thus: 'Some things for which we can give no reason are nevertheless manifest to the senses, while others which we perceive by no sense or sensation are manifest to the reason' (ii. 734). It is asserted that some facts must be accepted on a basis of observation tested by experiment, even though not accounted for by theory; conversely, some subjects can be explored only by reason (philosophy for example) because they cannot be tested by the objective criteria of the senses. The author goes on to discuss the necessity for observation and experiment, and the prime example of this, given in the next paragraph, is magnetic attraction. Aristotle (*Physics*, VIII. iv) said that the 'mover' must be in contact with the 'moved' for motion to result, which observation and experiment show is not true in this case. The *Libri Regimenti* again refers to the pseudo-Plato.

§ 20. The loadstone is the magnet. The Latin text includes also a reference to a stone which attracted straw, probably amber or pitch, which become charged with static electricity when rubbed; the 'certain other stone' may refer to a mineral (e.g. limestone) added in a metallurgical operation to 'draw' the slag ('glass') from the ore. 'After Plato' means 'according to [the pseudo-] Plato'.

phers to be in things by experience; which no man ought to deny [until it is tested] after the fashion of Philosophers which found [it].

For the Philosophers saith that the Palm is a tree, and it hath 21 the male and the female; therefore when the female is nigh the male, thou seest that the female bow down to the male, and the leaf and branches of it are made soft, and bow down to the male. Therefore when they see that, they bind ropes from the male to the female, *redit ergo erecta, super se ipsam quasi adepta sit masculo per continuationem funis virtutem masculi* [so it springs back upright, as if it has acquired from the male tree, through the connection of the rope, the virtue of the male]. Notwithstanding, many of the ancient authors hath shewed marvellous things, received now of the common people, and taken for a truth.

Therefore I shall show to thee certain things, that thou mayest 22 stablish thy mind upon them, and to know it for a certain truth which reason can not stablish by feeling, because the aforesaid help in them. And therefore it is, that the son of Messias said in the Book of the Beasts: if a woman great with child put on the apparel of a man, and a man put it on after, before he wash it, if he have the fever quartan, it will depart from him.

And it is said in the Book of Beasts that the Leopard fleeth 23

§ 21. From very ancient times male inflorescences of the Date Palm (*Phoenix dactylifera*) were tied into the crowns of the female trees to ensure a full crop of dates. Here it is the 'binding' which is thought to be significant, not the pollen. There follow nearly one hundred miscellaneous recipes, most of which appear to depend on sympathetic magic in one form or another. A number of conjuring tricks are also described.

§ 22. The son of Messias (Mesüe Junior, Masawijah al-Marindi, d. 1015) popularized the tradition of Arabian medicine in Latin translations. The author apparently discovered this saying of Mesüe Junior, and several subsequent recipes, in some kind of bestiary; the most popular 'book of beasts' in the Middle Ages was the 'Physiologus' (see Introduction, p. xxxvii), but this particular recipe is more likely to have come from the same source as Pliny's account (xxviii. 23. 82–3).

§ 23. *Cranium* ('skull') is a late Latin word not found in Elyot's dictionary;

the privy members of a man, and in another place it is said
si cranium of an old man be buried in a Dove or Culver house,
or be put where Doves or Culvers inhabit or rest, there they are
multiplied until it be full of them.

24   And in the book *De Tyriaca* of Galen, it is said that the

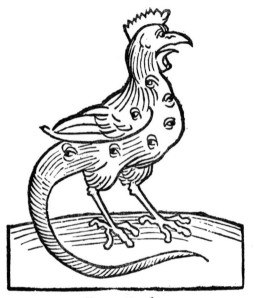

Fig. 29. Regulus.
From the *Hortus Sanitatis* (1491)

the translator, either guessing, or misled by a misprint, interpreted it as related
to *carnalis* or *carneus* 'carnal' or 'of the flesh', hence the reference to the 'privy
members' instead of 'skull', and the Latin phrase, which means 'if the skull . . .'

§ 24. No authentic work by Galen, a highly influential Greek physician of the
second century A.D., is known by the name *De Tyriaca* ('of antidotes'). The
fabulous cockatrice, often confused with the basilisk, has a fascinating history;
see T. H. White's *The Book of Beasts* (London, 1954), pp. 168 ff. Albertus
Magnus (*Animalia*, xxv. 13) wrote of the cockatrice, 'As to the statement that
a feeble old cock lays an egg and places it in dung; and that the egg has no shell
but only a skin so hard that it resists the hardest blows; and that the heat of the
sun hatches it into a basilisk, which is a serpent just like a cock in every way
except that it has the long tail of a serpent—I do not believe that this is true.
But Hermes says so, and many people accept it on his authority' (translated by
Wyckoff, p. 129). Two seasons of equal length are experienced in many sub-

Serpent which is called *Regulus* in Latin, a Cockatrice in English, is somewhat white, upon whose head there be three hairs, and when any man seeth them he dieth soon. And when any man or any other living thing heareth his whistling, he dieth. And every beast that eateth of it being dead, dieth also. And Aristotle said, where there is summer six months and likewise winter, there is a flood in the which Adders are found, whose property is that they never see themselves but they die; but when they be dead, they hurt not. And Aristotle put craftily in the mind of Alexander, that he should take a great glass and walk with it toward them, and when they did behold themselves in the glass they died. This saying of Aristotle was not believed of some men. For Avicenna said against Aristotle, if any man did see it, he died, wherefore there is no truth in his speech.

And they said, if any man would take of the milk of a 25 woman, giving suck to her own daughter of two year old, and let it be put in a glassen vessel, or hanged up in a Dove or Culver house where they go in and forth, Doves will abide and be multiplied there, until they be innumerable. And they said, when the mouth of a dead man is put upon him which complaineth of his belly, his belly is healed.

And Alexander said, when any thing is taken out of the 26 navel of an infant which cometh forth, if it be cut, and be put

tropical climates. Many stories of miraculous adventures concerning Alexander of Macedon circulated in the Middle Ages, and were attributed to Aristotle, who was the young king's tutor—see Introduction, p. xlii. A similar story is reported sceptically by Topsell as being a current 'old wives tale' in England (p. 681).

§ 25. The dove was regarded as a symbol of fecundity, and might be expected therefore to be capable of magically stimulating lactation in women; here, curiously, the reverse is asserted.

§ 26. 'Alexander' is here probably Alexander of Aphrodisias (fl. *c*. A.D. 200). Sorrel is *Rumex acetosa*; the leaves were formerly used to prepare a green sauce to be served with fish, and various decoctions used against fever. *Sepesquilla* is possibly squill (*Urginea maritima*), a medicinal herb with pungent aromatic bulbs, though 'squill' is usually rendered *Scilla* in Latin; *sepes* is Latin for hedge, but squill is not a hedgerow plant.

under the stone of a ring of silver or gold, then the passion or grief of the colic cometh not in any wise to him that beareth it.

And Galen saith, when the leaves of Sorrel be eaten, they loose the belly. And when the seed of it is drunken, it looseth the belly. And it is said that the root of Sorrel hanged upon him that hath the swine pox, it helpeth him.

And Philosophers say, when thou wilt that a beast return to his lodging, anoint his forehead with *Sepesquilla*, and it will return.

27   And Aristotle said, in the Book of the Beasts, if any man put wrought wax upon the horns of [a] Cow's Calf, it will go with him wheresoever he will, without labour. And if any man anoint the horn of Kine with wax and oil or pitch the pain of their feet goeth away.

And if any shall anoint the tongues of Oxen with any tallow, they [will] neither taste nor eat meat, but they shall die for hunger, except it be wiped away with salt and vinegar.

And if any man anoint the nether parts of a Cock with oil, he neither will, nor may tread an Hen.

If thou desire that a Cock crow not, anoint his head and forehead with oil.

It is said in the book of Archigenis *quando cavilla* [when an ankle] of the Hare is hanged upon him that suffereth the colic, it profiteth him.

And Aristotle said the haemorrhoids goeth away from him, which sitteth upon the skin of a Lion.

And if the dung of an Hare be broken unto powder and cast abroad upon a place of Emmets, or Pismires, then the Pismires leave their place.

28   Philosophers said, if the head of a Goat be hanged upon him

§ 27. The lion's skin as a cure for haemorrhoids is mentioned by Topsell (p. 378), and attributed by him to Galen; in the *Hortus Sanitatis* (p. 51), however, the source is given as Aesculapius. 'Emmets' or 'pismires' are ants. The reference to Aristotle again comes from a work falsely ascribed to him; for a discussion of the sources cited in this section, see the Introduction, pp. xli–xlii.

§ 28. The wolf is associated with the prevention of lechery in two other recipes

which suffereth swine pox, he is healed by it. If thou wilt that a woman be not vitiate nor desire men, take the privy member of a Wolf, and the hairs which do grow on the cheeks or eye bright of him, and the hairs which be under his beard, and burn it all, and give it to her in a drink when she knoweth not, and she shall desire no other man. And they said, when a woman desireth not her husband, then let her husband take a little of the tallow of a buck Goat, mean between little and great, and let him anoint his privy member with it, and do the act of generation; she shall love him and shall not do the act of generation afterward with any [other].

And they said that when the Snail is poisoned, it eateth the herb called Origanum, and is healed, and therefore they know that the herb called Origanum hath lain under poison. Also it is said when the Weasel is poisoned of a Serpent it eateth Rue, and they know by this that Rue is contrary to the venom of Serpents.

And a Mouse, put under the pricking of Scorpions, delivereth a man because she is contrary and feareth not him.

And Philosophers have invented that if any woman is barren, when there is put to her a thing that maketh a woman barren, that woman is not barren, but fruitful, and contrariwise.

And it is said that when a Sponge is cast in wine mixed with water and after drawn forth and strained and wringed, the water cometh forth of it, and the wine remaineth. If it be not mixed, nothing cometh forth.

—see pp. 58 and 91. 'Eye bright' is a variant of 'eye bree' meaning 'eyelid'. The goat was regarded as a symbol of sexual virility; but a little of any tallow would probably be effective. The translator has omitted a number of other recipes of a similar nature.

§ 29. These two statements come unchanged from Pliny (viii. 41. 98); the 'snail' again refers to the tortoise. *Origanum vulgare* is marjoram or organy; rue or 'herb of grace' is *Ruta graveolens*.

§ 30. This is an extension, almost a contradiction, of the principle of affinity, presumably by the logic that two negatives make a positive.

31   Tabariensis said, if a stone be hanged upon a Sponge, on the neck of a child which cougheth with a vehement or great cough, his cough is mitigated and restrained. And when it is put on the head of an Ass, or into his fundament, *Scarabeus*

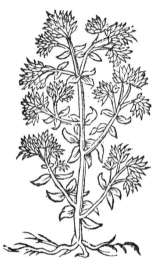

Fig. 30. *Origanum*, organy.
From *Naturalia Alberti Magni* (1548)

(that is a fly with a black shell, that breedeth in cowshards and is black, called a Beetle) cutteth him and he turneth, until it be drawn from him.

It is said also, that if any stone be bounden to the tail of an Ass, he will not bray nor roar.

32   If the hairs of an Ass be taken, which are nigh his privy member, and be given to any man broken in with any kind of wine in a drink, he beginneth anon to fart. Likewise if any man taketh the eggs of Pismires and breaketh them, and casteth them

§ 31. The last suggestion would probably have the effect indicated. The insect intended is one of the dung beetles, of which the commonest is *Geotrupes stercorarius*, here subsumed under the name of the Egyptian sacred scarab beetle (*Ateuchus sacer*). The explanatory parenthesis is taken from Elyot's dictionary.

§ 32. 'Pismires' are ants, and the 'eggs' are no doubt the pupae of the insect, still sold in pet shops as an aquarium fish food.

into water, and give them to any man in a drink, he ceaseth not anon to fart. They do likewise with wine.

And it is said, if thou wilt make a ring of a rod of a fresh 33 Myrtle tree, and put it on thy ring finger, it mitigateth or extincteth the impostume under the arm holes.

In the book of Aristotle, it is said that the root of white Henbane, when it is hanged upon a man suffering the colic, it is profitable to him. And when Saltpetre is put in a vessel, and vinegar upon it, it will boil or seethe mightily without fire.

It is said also in the book of Hermes, when Leek seed is casten upon vinegar, the eagerness or sourness of it goeth away.

Belbinus said, when thou takest the white of an egg and 34 Alum and anointeth a cloth with it, and washest it off with water of the sea, being dry, it letteth the fire to burn.

Another said, when red *Arsenicum* and Alum are taken, and broken, and confected, or made with the juice of the herb called Houseleek, and the gall of a Bull, and a man anointeth his hand with it, and after taketh hot Iron, it burneth not them. Likewise if there be taken *ex Magne*, and Alum *jamenti*, and strong vinegar, and Great Mallows or Hollyhock, if thou bray them well together and anoint thy hands therewith, fire hurtethnot them.

When thou wilt that they which be in a palace seem without

§ 33. A 'rod' is a twig, and 'impostumes' are boils or abscesses. White 35 henbane is *Hyoscyamus albus*, a larger plant with more attractive flowers than common henbane, *H. niger* (see under *Jusquiamus*, p. 10). 'Saltpetre' (potassium nitrate) is clearly a mistranslation of the more general word *salsum* in the Latin text; the salt referred to is sodium carbonate. This recipe gives instructions for a perfectly feasible conjuring trick, recorded also by Sir Hugh Platt in *The Jewell-house of Art and Nature* (1594) p. 31.

§ 34. Again 'letteth' is used in the sense 'preventeth'. Red arsenic is realgar, the red sulphide of arsenic (As_2S_2), and *magne* is magnetite (magnetic iron oxide, Fe_2O_3). The Latin word *jamenti* is obscure; elsewhere it is translated as 'bitter' alum. Several sets of instructions for carrying out conjuring tricks involving noninflammability are given. The essential ingredients are (i) alum, mixed with (ii) a viscous fluid—egg-white, or the juices of mucilaginous plants such as houseleek (*Sempervivum tectorum*) and hollyhock (*Althaea rosea*). See the summary, in the text, of the substances which 'have virtue in this matter', p. 108.

§ 35. The phrase 'smart brimstone' reads as if it might imply 'molten', but probably signifies 'native', or naturally occurring sulphur. Common purslane

heads, take smart Brimstone, with oil, and put it in a lamp and make light with it, and put it in the midst of men, and thou shalt see a marvellous thing.

And Belbinus said again, he that shall put an herb called Purslane upon his bed shall not see dream nor vision utterly.

And Aristotle saith, that Mares when they smell the smoke of a lamp put out, they bring forth their birth before it be perfect, and likewise this chanceth to certain women with child.

36   Aristotle said, that if any man causeth by his wit a Camel to do the act of generation with his own mother, if he perceive it before, he will pursue the man until he kill him. And if he cause by his wit an Horse to leap his own mother, and he know it before, he will kill himself and him that provoked him to that.

37   And Philosophers saith, if thou drown Flies in the water, they seem dead, and if they be buried in ashes, they rise up again. And when thou drownest *Aomber*, it dieth, and let vinegar be dropped down like dew upon it, it is quickened. And when thou buryest the fly called a Beetle among roses, it dieth; if thou bury it in dung, it quickeneth.

38   And Philosophers said that when the feathers of Eagles be

is *Portulaca oleracea*, low-growing succulent plants used as a potherb, and as a herbal remedy for 'cooling the blood'.

§ 36. The *Hortus Sanitatis* records, somewhat more circumstantially, the same anecdote of the camel: '. . . and though the camel be uncleanly and foul in his works, yet he is very cleanly towards his dame, as it hath been proved in a great lord's court that there was once a camel disposed to the works of nature and to her was brought one of her own young, and her head was wound in a clout [cloth] because that her young should not know her. Thus engendering not knowing each other they were left together . . . Then was the female's head unbound and the young seeing that he had engendered with his dame, he did make great heaviness and mourning manners as one being sore ashamed of the deed, and bit off his yard or member and so slew himself; which to us is a great example' (p. 29). The common source is probably Aelian (iii. 47).

§ 37. The same experiment with flies is reported above on p. 9; if this account is taken from the same source, *aomber* (from *bombus*?) may be bees. Various beetles burrow into dung and flourish there, but death from roses is more likely to be symbolic than actual.

§ 38. The feathers of the eagle have the same general power as the skin of a

put with the feathers of other fowls they burn and mortify them; for as he overcometh in his life all birds, and ruleth over them, so the feathers of Eagles are deadly to all feathers.

And Philosophers say, if the skin of a Sheep be put in any place with the skin of *Adib*, it gnaweth and consumeth it. And he that putteth on him cloth of the wool of a Sheep which hath eaten *Adib*, itching ceaseth not from him until he put it off.

And if thou perfume an house or place with the lungs or lights of an Ass, thou cleanest it from every Serpent and Scorpion. And of this Philosophers know that it is good against poison.

Tabariensis saith, if the tongue of the Lapwing or Black Plover be hanged upon a wall *oblivionem redit cum memorem et alienationes*.

And it is said in the book of Cleopatra, if a woman have no 39 delectation with her husband, take the marrow of a Wolf, of his left foot, and bear it, and she will love no man but him. And it is said, when the left hip or haunch of a male Ostrich is taken and boiled, or seethed with oil, and after, the beginning or ground of hairs are anointed with it, they grow never again.

Architas said, if the heart of a Serpent be taken when he liveth, and be hanged upon a man, being sick of the fever quartan, it plucketh it utterly away. And the Adder's skin, when it is strait bounden upon the ankle of a woman, it

---

wolf (see p. 76). Thomas Lupton (ii. 70) translates Aelian (ix. 2) on this subject: 'The quills or pens of an Eagle, mixed with the quills or pens of other fowls or birds, doth consume or waste them with their odour, smell, or air.' *Adib* remains obscure. The Latin phrase may be translated 'it causes loss of consciousness, [loss of] memory, and delirium'. Of the hoopoe, mistranslated as the lapwing, the *Hortus Sanitatis* records, 'whoso is anointed with his blood shall have many devilish fantasies' (p. 125).

§ 39. The wolf is credited with the power to remove lechery from both man and woman (see above, pp. 58 and 87). The serpent, the phallic symbol *par excellence*, has been regarded as life- and health-giving since earliest times, and in the form of the Aesculapian snake (*Elaphe longissima*) is still the emblem of the medical profession. The slough of a snake, a perfect replica of itself cast off whole from the living animal, is a symbol of rebirth, and thought to be efficacious in easing childbirth.

hasteth the birth, but after the birth, it must be removed away anon.

40   The teeth of all Serpents, when thou pluckest them forth by the roots, as long as the Serpent liveth, if they be hanged upon a man, sick of the fever quartan, they take away the fever quartan from him, and if the Serpent be hanged upon a tooth aching it profiteth. And if a Serpent meet with a woman with child, she bringeth forth her child before it be perfect. And if it meet with her when she travaileth of child, it hasteth her birth.

41   And they say, if thou wilt take the eye tooth of the beast called *Crocodilus* in Latin, in English a Crocodile, out of the uppermore palate of the left side of his mouth, and hang it on a man being sick of the fevers, it healeth him and the fevers will not return again to him. And they have said that the Lion is afraid of a white Cock. And again that he feareth the fire. And he that is anointed with the tallow of the reins of the Lion, feareth not to go among beasts, and all beasts are afraid of the Lion. And he that anointeth his body with Hare's dung, Wolves be afraid of him.

42   *Et si teritur arsenicum citrinum* [and if yellow Arsenic be brayed] and be mixed with milk, if a Fly fall upon it, it dieth.

§ 40. The fangs of venomous snakes, being poisonous, were thought to be effective against the poison of fever; here the magic is attributed to all snakes. The power of snakes to cause abortion when merely encountered was put to the test (with negative results) as late as 1669 by M. Charas (*New Experiments with Vipers*).

§ 41. The crocodile, a large 'serpent', has the same magical qualities attributed to the snake in the previous paragraph. The lion being afraid of a white cock is mentioned above (p. 80) and is taken from Pliny. The *Hortus Sanitatis* reports, 'He that is anointed with the suet . . . of the kidney ('reins') of the noble lion, the wolves shall be of him right sore adread' (p. 51). Topsell records a different use for hare's dung: 'Whereas it was no small honour to Virgins in ancient time, to have their breasts continually stand out, every one was prescribed to drink in Wine or such other things, nine grains of Hare's dung' (p. 217).

§ 42. Yellow arsenic is orpiment (*auri pigmentum*, As_2S_3), from which Albertus Magnus prepared metallic arsenic by heating it with soap. The 'snail' is a tortoise; 'a man that is brosten' means a man who has a hernia; 'stones' are testicles, and 'bouncing' is used in the older sense of a sharp noise.

If thou wilt take the right foot of a Snail, and hang it upon the right foot of a diseased man with the gout, it profiteth it. Likewise if thou hang up the left foot of a Snail to thy left foot, diseased with the gout. And so the hand of it is profitable to the hand and the finger to the finger. And if a fire of green wood of Fig trees be kindled before a man that is brosten, his stones will make a noise or bouncing.

And it is said in the book of Hermes, when both the eyes 43 of the Bear be bounden in linen cloth, upon *sinistrum adiutorium*, they put away the fever quartan. And it is said, if the Wolf see a man and the man see not him, the man is astonished and feareth, and is hoarse. And therefore if any man beareth the eye of a Wolf, it helpeth to victory, to boldness, vanquishing, and fear in his adversary. And it is said, if a ring be made of the white hoofs of an Ass, and he that hath the falling sickness putteth it on, [he] suffereth not the falling sickness.

And they said, when thou wilt that Flies come not nigh thy 44 house, then put *Condisum et Opium* in white Lime, and after make thy house white with it, then Flies shall in no wise enter.

When thou wilt that thy wife or wench show to thee all that she hath done, take the heart of a Dove and the head of a Frog, and dry them both, and bray them unto powder, and lay them upon the breast of her sleeping, and she shall show to thee all that she hath done; but when she shall wake, wipe it away from her breast, that she be not lifted up.

And they say, if any man put a Diamond under the head 45

§ 43. The Latin phrase probably means '[upon] the left side, they help'. The *Hortus Sanitatis* is more informative about 'man meets wolf': 'If the wolf see the man first, then taketh he from man his voice because he should not cry, as one that were of the wolf overcome; but if the man see the wolf first then the wolf loseth thereby his courage and also is pale that he cannot run' (p. 55).

§ 44. *Condisum* is black hellebore (*Helleborus niger*) and *opium* the opium poppy (*Papaver somniferum*); both plants are sources of powerful narcotic drugs. The 'truth drug' effect may be attributed more to the head of the frog than the heart of the dove; see p. 99 below, where the sympathetic magic is more obvious. The phrase 'that she be not lifted up' might better have been translated 'that she become not delirious' (*ne alienetur*).

§ 45. The test of fidelity is described above (p. 26) with a magnet rather than

of a woman sleeping, she manifesteth if she be an adulterer, for if it be so, she leapeth back out of the bed afraid, and if not, she embraceth her husband with great love.

And they say that an Ass skin when it is hanged upon children, it letteth them to be afraid.

Architas saith, if the wax of the left ear of a Dog be taken, and be hanged upon men sick in the fevers that come by course or fits, it is very profitable, and specially to the fever quartan.

And Philosophers say that some kind or singular, which never had sickness, is profitable to every sickness; and he that had never pain, helpeth and healeth a man from it.

And when the house is perfumed with the left hoof of a Mule, Flies remain not in it.

46   And if the heart, eye or brain of a Lapwing or Black Plover be hanged upon a man's neck, it is profitable against forget﹣fulness, and sharpeth man's understanding.

If a woman may not conceive take an Hart's horn, turned into powder, and let it be mixed with a Cow's gall, let a woman keep it about her, and let her do the act of generation, and she shall conceive anon.

A gross and stiff hair of a Mare's tail, put upon a door suffereth not *Zinzalas* to enter.

The tooth of a Foal or Colt of one year old, put in the neck of a child, maketh his teeth to breed without pain.

The tooth of a Mare put upon the head of a man, being mad, delivereth him anon from his fury.

47   If a woman may not conceive, let a Mare's milk be given to

a diamond; Wyckoff (p. 71) describes the ancient confusion between the properties of these two stones. The phrase 'kind or singular' means 'species or individual' (see above, p. 75).

§ 46. The *Hortus Sanitatis* reports of the hoopoe (consistently mistranslated as 'lapwing', see p. 56 above) that 'The tongue of it hanged on one that is very forgetful, it shall keep him in good remembrance' (p. 125). Powdered hart's horn as an aphrodisiac in Europe is paralleled by the powdered rhinoceros horn still valued in Asia. '*Zinzalas*' are gnats.

§ 47. The translator has omitted many recipes both to promote conception and to prevent it. The *Hortus Sanitatis* appears to be quoting this work when it

her not knowing, let her do the act of generation in that hour, and she shall conceive anon.

The hoof of an Horse perfumed in a house, driveth away Mice. The same chanceth also by the hoof of a Mule.

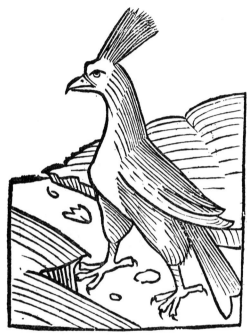

FIG. 31. *Upupa*, the hoopoe, as the woodcut shows, is a crested bird; the fact that the lapwing is also crested probably led to the confusion between the two birds. From the *Hortus Sanitatis* (1491)

That all the hot water come forth of a cauldron. Take of 48 blanch, that is *Terra francisca*, with pitch; cast it in water, and

records: 'Albertus saith make a smoke in your house of the left hoof of a mule and all the rats shall run away' (p. 67).

§ 48. The reaction of water with lime would certainly generate much heat, and possibly the heated sulphur might catch fire on exposure to air. Small pieces of camphor float on water and move about, but do not catch fire. It is of course not a herb in the sense of a herbaceous plant, but the product of a tree (*Cinnamomum camphora*) from the wood or young shoots of which it is steam-distilled.

it shall come forth all. That fire may come forth of water, take the shell of an egg and put in it quick Brimstone and Lime, and shut the hole and put it into water and it will kindle.

And it is said, if the herb Camphor be put upon water, it is kindled and burneth in the water.

49   That thou may take birds with thy hands, take any corn very well steeped in the dregs of wine and in the juice of Hemlock and cast it to the birds. Every bird that tasteth of it is made drunken, and loseth her strength.

And they say if any man be anointed with the milk of an Ass all the Flies of the house will gather to him.

To write letters or bills, which be not read but in the night. Take the gall of a Snail or milk of a Sow, and put it to the fire, or with water of a worm shining late.

If ye mingle together many whites of Hens' eggs, a month after, they are made glass, and hard as a stone, and of this being after this fashion is made a sophistical precious stone, called *Topazos*, if it be conjoined before with saffron or red earth.

50   Likewise, if the foam which is found about the stones of an Hart or Horse, or Ass, being weary, be mixed with wine, and the wine be given to any man to drink, he shall abhor wine for a month.

And if any man shall have many Eels in a wine vessel, and

§ 49. These recipes would probably be effective. Almost any liquid containing organic matter will do as crude 'invisible ink'. The writing can only be read with difficulty until exposed to heat, when it darkens. The glow-worm is the larva of a beetle (*Lampyris noctiluca*). Sir Hugh Platt (*The Jewell-house of Art and Nature*, 1594, p. 13) was aware of the same phenomenon when he wrote 'How to write a letter secretly that cannot easily be discovered, or suspected. Write your mind at large on the one side of the paper with common ink, and on the other side with milk that which you would have secret, and when you would make the same legible, hold that side which is written with ink to the fire, and the milky letters will show bluish on the other side.' The last paragraph is a somewhat garbled version of a recipe for making a 'paste' semi-precious stone.

§ 50. After this paragraph the nature of the marvels changes somewhat; many of the 'perfumings' which follow appear to have originated in the work of Marcus Grecus, the *Book of Fires*. The undoubted effect of certain hallucinogenic vegetable drugs if perfumed in a lamp has been extended to various kinds of sympathetic magic.

they be suffered to die in it, if any man drink of it, he shall abhor wine for a year, and by chance evermore.

And it is said, if a rope be taken, with which a thief is or hath been hanged up, and a little chaff, which a whirlwind lifted up in the air, and let them be put in a pot, and set among other pots, that pot shall break all the other pots.

Also take thou a little of the aforesaid rope, and put it on the instrument with which the bread is put in the oven; when he that should put it in the oven, should put it in, he shall not be able to put it in, but it shall leap out.

That men may seem without heads. 51

Take an Adder's skin and *auri pigmentum*, and Greek pitch and *Reuponticum*, and the wax of new Bees, and the fat or grease of an Ass, and break them all, and put them in a dull seething pot full of water, and make it to seethe at a slow fire, and after let it wax cold, and make a taper, and every man that shall see light of it shall seem headless.

That men may seem to have the visage or countenance of a Dog.

Take the fat out of the ear of a Dog, and anoint with it a little new silk, put it in a new lamp of green glass, and put the lamp among men, and they shall see the visage of a Dog.

That men may seem to have three heads.

Take the hair of a dead Ass, and make a rope, and dry it, and take the marrow of the principal bone of his right shoulder, and mix it with virgin wax, and anoint the cord, and put it upon the lamps of the house; they that come into the house shall

§ 51. *Auri pigmentum* is orpiment, arsenic trisulphide (As_2S_3). *Reu ponticum* or *reu barbarum* is rhubarb; the medicinal plant used by herbalists is *Rheum officinale*, and the culinary plant *R. rhaponticum*.

seem to have three heads, and they that be in the house shall seem Asses to them that enter in.

52   If thou wilt that a man's head
                           seem an Ass head.

Take up of the covering of an Ass and anoint the man on his head.

53   If thou wilt that a Chicken or other
                           thing leap in the dish.

Take Quicksilver and the powder of Calamine, and put it in a bottle of glass well spotted and put it within an hot thing. For seeing Quicksilver is hot, it moveth itself, and maketh it to leap or dance.

                   If thou wilt see that other men can not.

Take of the gall of a male Cat, and the fat of an Hen all white, and mix them together, and anoint thy eyes, and thou shalt see it that others can not see.

54   If thou wilt understand the
                           voices of birds.

Associate with thee two fellows in the twenty-eighth day of October, and go into a certain wood with Dogs as to hunt,

§ 52. 'Covering' mistranslates the Latin *segimine*, 'fat'; apparently the translator's text had *tegimine* 'a cover'.

§ 53. Calamine is zinc carbonate. The phrase 'well spotted' translates the Latin *sigillatam*, which refers to the common practice of using special designs and images as a part of the magical procedure. Thomas Lupton (x. 33) reports a similar property of quicksilver: 'Take a ring that is hollow round about, into which put quicksilver, and stop the same fast, that it run not forth; after heat the ring somewhat in the fire, which being hot, lay on a table or stool and soon after it will leap or dance of itself until it be cold. It is Proved.'

§ 54. The Latin original of this passage is made the starting-point of an amusing anecdote in the ironical work *Beware the Cat* (1561) by William Baldwin, where the narrator elaborates on the ritual suggested in outline here, and does eventually learn to understand the voices of birds (ed. William P. Holden, 1963, pp. 40 ff.).

and carry home with [thee] that beast which thou shalt find first, and prepare it with the heart of a Fox, and thou shalt understand anon the voice of birds or beasts. And if thou wilt that any other likewise understand, kiss him, and he shall understand.

If thou wilt loose bonds.   55

Go into the wood, and look where the Pie hath her nest with her birds, and when thou shalt be there, climb up the tree, and bind about the hole of it wheresoever thou wilt. For when she seeth thee, she goeth for a certain herb, which she will put to the binding, and it is broken anon and that herb falleth to the ground upon the cloth, which thou shouldst have put under the tree, and be thou present and take it.

That a man may be always as a gelded man.

Take of the worm, which shineth in summer, and give it to him to drink.

That a woman may confess   56
what she hath done.

Take a water Frog quick, and take away her tongue, and put it again into the water, and put the tongue unto a part of the

§ 55. The herb used by the magpie may be mistletoe (see pp. 12–13). The stone found in the nest of the 'lapwing' is *quiritia* (p. 41), but the description here better fits *ophthalmus* (p. 26).

§ 56. Topsell, quoting the *Kiranides*, records more fully, and more sceptically, the same magical power of the frog: 'If he will know the secrets of woman, then must he cut the tongue out of the Frog alive, and turn the Frog away again, making certain characters upon the Frog's tongue, and so lay the same upon the panting of a woman's heart, and let him ask her what questions he will, she shall answer unto him all the truth, and reveal all the secret faults that ever she had committed. Now if this magical foolery were true, we had more need of Frogs than of Justices of the Peace or Magistrates in the Commonwealth' (p. 723).

heart of the woman sleeping, which when she is asked, she shall say the truth.

**If thou wilt put any man in
fear in his sleep.**

Put under his head the skin of an Ape.

57

If thou wilt take a Mole.

Put in his hole an Onion, or a Leek or Garlic and she will come soon forth without strength.

A Serpent goeth not nigh Garlic, and a Dog tasteth not any thing dipped with Garlic, although he be hungry.

58

**A perfuming by which every man shall seem to
other that be in the house, in the form of
Elephants and great Horses.**

Take a spice which is called *Alcachengi*, and bray it, mix it with a little fat of a Dolphin fish, and make thereof grains, as be of *Pomecitron*. After, perfume some of them upon a fire of Cow's dung, which is milked. And let not a place be in the house, from which smoke may come forth, but the gate, and let the fire be under the earth within; all which be in the lodging, shall seem as they were great men in the shape of Horses and Elephants, and it is a very marvellous thing.

§ 57. Thomas Hill in *The Profitable Arte of Gardening* (1593) reports: 'And Albertus writeth, that if you stop the holes of Moles with either Garlic, Onions or Leeks, that any of these, do either force him forthwith to run from that place, or to cast up anew in some other place' (p. 33).

§ 58. *Alcachengi* is the winter cherry (*Physalis alkekengi*), and the mixture should be made into little balls ('grains') the size of lemon ('*pomecitron*') pips.

Another perfuming, which when thou makest,   59
thou seest outwardly green men, and men of
many shapes and infinite marvels which are
not discerned for their multitude.

Take *Timar*, that is Vermilion, and the stone *Lazulus* and
Pennyroyal of the mountains and beat it all to powder, and

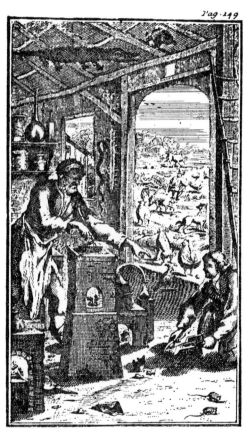

Pag. 149

FIG. 32. An experimenter, presumably Albertus Magnus, works with the dung
of various animals, while a disciple collects specimens.
From *Les Admirables Secrets d'Albert le Grand* (1758)

§ 59. Vermilion, a permanent bright red pigment, mercuric sulphide, is

sift it. Mix it with the fat of a Dolphin fish, Horse or Elephant, make grains or corns after the fashion of Rice, and dry them in a shadow. Perfume in it when thou wilt and it shall be done that is said.

60   A perfuming to see in our sleep what thing
                    is to come of good and evil.

Take the blood of an Ass congealed, and the fat *Lupi Cervini*, and a sweet incense or gum called *storax* and also *styrax*; gather it all together by equal weights and let them be mixed, and grains or corns be made thereof, and let the house be perfumed with them, that thou shalt see him in thy sleep that shall shew to thee all things.

61   A manner of making a match of a candle, or
              candle wick, which when thou shalt kindle,
                 thou shalt see men in what shape soever
                              thou wilt.

Take the eyes of a Shriek Owl, the eyes of a fish, which is called *Affures*, and the eyes of a fish, which is called *Libinitis*, and the gall of Wolves; break them with thy hands, and mix them together, and put them in a vessel of glass. Then when thou wilt work it, take the fat of any beast thou wilt, that this may be made in the shape of it, melt it, and mix it perfectly with that medicine, and anoint the match or candle wick, whatsoever thou wilt, with it. After, kindle it in the midst of the house, and the men shall seem in the shape of that beast whose fat thou didst take.

purified from the mineral cinnabar by sublimation. Lazuli is an aluminium silicate mineral which forms the basis of the bright blue pigment ultramarine. 'Pennyroyal of the mountains' may be *Veronica montana* (speedwell); true penny-royal is *Mentha pulegium*.

§ 60. *Lupi Cervini* is 'of a wolf [or] of a deer'; storax (or styrax) is the resin from the gum tree *Liquidambar orientalis*.

§ 61. For the shriek owl, see p. 52, where it is associated with a 'truth drug' effect. The fish have not been identified.

Another match of a candle or a candle wick,   62
that men may appear in the shape of angels.

Take the eyes of a fish, and the eyes of *Filoe*, that is of a breaker
of bones, and break them with thy hands, and make them soft,
and put them in a vessel of glass seven days. After, put some
oil in them, and lighten it in a green lamp, and put it before
men which be in the house; they shall see themselves in the
shape of angels by the light of the fire.

Another match or wick of a candle, making   63
men to appear with black faces.

Take a black lamp, and pour in it oil of the Elder or Alder
tree, or Quicksilver, and pour in that oil or Quicksilver a
part of the blood of them that be in letting blood, and put in
that blood oil of the Elder or Alder tree (some saith of the Bur
tree) or Quicksilver.

A marvellous lamp, in which appeareth
a thing of terrible quantity, having
in the hand a rod, and affrayeth a man.

Take a green Frog, and strike off the head of it upon a green
cloth, make it wet with the oil of Bur tree or Elder tree, and
put in the wick and lighten it in the green lamp; then shalt

§ 62. *Filoe* seems to be a corruption of the Greek *phenes*, an osprey (*Pandion
haliaetus*). The Latin name of the osprey, *ossifragus*, is explained in the *Kiranides*
(1685, p. 126) as 'a bird that breaks bones . . . for it does not only eat flesh,
but the very bones'.

§ 63. Alder (*Alnus glutinosa*) is a tree of magical importance in Celtic folklore,
partly perhaps because the wood when cut shows white, and then turns bright
red. Elder (*Sambucus nigra*) is a quite different plant, a vigorous shrub rather
than a tree, regarded as magic from very early times (it provided the timber for
the True Cross, and Judas hanged himself on it), used medicinally by the
ancient Egyptians, and officinal in Britain as late as 1949. Turner (1548) gives
'Boure tree' as an alternative English name, and it is still called 'bour-tree' in
the north of England.

thou see a black man standing, between whose hands there shall be a lamp and a marvellous thing.

64   Another wick which when it is kindled, and
water is poured on it, waxeth strong, and
when the oil is put in, it is put out.

Take Lime which water hath not touched and put it with a weight equal to it of wax, and the half of it of the oil of Balm and *Naphtha citrina*, with equal to it of Brimstone, and make a wick of it, and drop the water down like dew upon it and it shall be kindled, and drop down oil upon it, and it shall be put out.

Another wick, which when it is kindled,
all things seem white and of silver.

Take a Lizard and cut away the tail of it, and take that which cometh out, for it is like Quicksilver. After, take a wick and make it wet with oil, and put it in a new lamp and kindle it, and the house shall seem bright and white, or gilded with silver.

A marvellous operation of a lamp, which
if any man shall hold, he ceaseth not to
fart until he shall leave it.

Take the blood of a Snail, dry it up in a linen cloth, and make of it a wick, and lighten it in a lamp, give it to any man thou wilt, and say lighten this, he shall not cease to fart, until he let it depart, and it is a marvellous thing.

§ 64. Balm is the aromatic herb *Melissa officinalis*, but the oil mentioned here is probably the secretion of the 'Balm of Gilead tree', *Cemmiphora opobalsamum*. Naphtha is the inflammable liquid fraction of naturally occurring bitumen; the commoner sorts are tinged yellow (*citrina*), but that which comes from certain deposits in the area of the Caspian Sea is water-white. This conjuring trick could probably be made to work (see note, p. 95).

A wick which when it is lightened, women   65
cease not to dance and be glad and to
play as they were mad for great joy.

Take the blood of an Hare and the blood of a certain fowl
which is called *Solon*, and is like a Turtle Dove, and of the
blood of the Turtle male, equal to the half of it. Then put in
it a wick, and lighten it in the midst of the house, in which
are singers and wenches, and a marvellous thing shall be
proved.

If thou wilt make that Lice may appear   66
running abroad in a man's bed that he
may not sleep.

Then cast in his bed the weight of [an] ounce, or half ounce of
Alcachengi. And if thou shalt take *pilos Asturis*, thereof shall be
made a wick, which when it is lightened, every sick man seeth
other by the vehemency of the sickness, and minishing or
extenuation.

When thou wilt that thou seem all inflamed,   67
or set on fire from thy head unto thy feet
and not be hurt.

Take white Great Mallows or Hollyhock, mix them with the
white of eggs; after, anoint thy body with it, and let it be until
it be dried up, and after anoint thee with Alum, and afterward
cast on it small Brimstone beaten unto powder, for the fire is
inflamed on it, and hurteth not, and if thou do thus upon the
palm of thy hand thou shalt be able to hold the fire without hurt.

§ 65. *Solon* is a gannet (*Sula bassana*); for the turtle dove see above, p. 58.

§ 66. Winter cherry (*Physalis alkekengi*) seems to be used here as some sort of
itching powder. The feathers of a hawk ('*pilos Asturis*'), possibly the goshawk
(*Accipiter gentilis*), are credited with the power of producing hallucinations in
sick people, of a strength determined by the degree of fever.

§ 67. 'Great mallows' is another name for hollyhock. See note, p. 89.

If thou wilt that a thing be casten
in the fire and not burn.

Take one part of glue of fish and an equal quantity to it of Alum, let it be perfectly mixed, and let vinegar be poured upon it; let whatsoever thing thou wilt, be confected with it to be cast in the fire, anoint it with this anointment, it shall not be burned.

68

If thou wilt make a contrary, that is any
image or other thing, and when it is put in
the water it is kindled, and if thou shalt
draw it out, it shall be put out or quenched.

Take Lime not quenched, and mix it perfectly with a little wax and the oil of *Sesamum*, and Naphtha, that is white earth, and Brimstone, and make of it an image. When thou shalt put it in water, the fire shall be kindled.

69

If thou wilt make that when thou openest thy
hands upon a lamp, the light of it is put out,
and when thou closest them upon it, it kindleth,
and it ceaseth not to do that.

Take a spice, which is called *Spuma*, after bray it, and after make it with water of Camphor, and anoint thy hands with it. After, open them in the mouth of the lamp; the light of it shall be put out, and close them and it shall be kindled again.

§ 68. See the note after a similar recipe, p. 104. The additional ingredient, oil of sesame, is the edible oil obtained from the seeds of *Sesamum indicum*. The mention of an 'image' suggests a connection with witchcraft.

§ 69. *Spuma* may be saponin, a foaming agent obtained from the herb *Saponaria officinalis*. For camphor, see note, p. 95.

If thou wilt see a thing drowned, or see   70
deep in the water in the night, and that it
shall not be more hid to thee than in the
day, and read books in a dark night.

Anoint thy face with the blood of the Rearmouse or Bat, and
it shall be done that I say. If thou wilt make any thing white
perfume it with Brimstone.

If thou wilt kill soon a Serpent.   71

Take as much as thou wilt of an herb called *Rotunda Aristologia*,
Smerwort, or Meek Galingale and bray it well, and take a
Frog of the wood or field and break it well, and mix it with
Aristologia, and put it with some ink and write with [it] in
paper or in any other thing which thou lovest better, and cast
it to Serpents.

If thou wilt bear fire in thy hand,   72
that it may not hurt thee.

Take Lime, dissolved with hot water of Beans, and a little
Magrencules, and a little of Great Mallows or Hollyhock, and
mix it well with it. After, anoint the palm of thy hand with it,
and let it be dried; put in it fire, and it shall not hurt.

§ 70. The bat (also called 'rearmouse') can, of course, 'see' in the dark, hence
its sympathetic magic. The fumes of burning sulphur (i.e. sulphur dioxide)
have a strong bleaching effect.

§ 71. Turner (1548) calls *Aristolochia rotunda* 'heartwort', and says it is confused
by some with 'holewort' (*Corydalis bulbosa*); both plants have round tubers, but
in the latter they are hollow. 'Galingale' is the aromatic tuber of *Alpinia offici-
narum*, formerly used as a substitute for ginger. *The Book of Medicines* (ed. and
trans. Sir E. A. T. W. Budge in *Syrian Anatomy, Pathology and Therapeutics*,
London, 1913), a work of the 'early centuries of the Christian Era' (p. v),
records: 'Whosoever burneth a frog, and scattereth its ashes about a house,
from that house serpents shall flee.'

§ 72. '*Magrencules*' is unidentified; it just might be *ranunculus* (buttercup).
Since the salamander was thought to live in fire, its blood would naturally be
thought immune from the effects of heat.

Philosophers say that such Lime burneth not in the fire. And glue of fish saveth from fire, and unpleasant Alum, and the blood of the beast called Salamander, and the smoke of an oven or cauldron. Therefore when an anointment is made of all these or of certain of them, the fire hurteth not. The

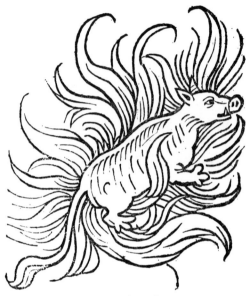

FIG. 33. *Salamandra.*
From the *Hortus Sanitatis* (1491)

white of an egg, and Great Mallows or Hollyhock have virtue in this matter.

A wick which when it is lightened in the
house, thou shalt see green things flying
as Sparrows and other birds.

Take a new cloth and put in it the brains of a bird, and the feathers of her tail, and lap them in, and make a wick of them, and put it in a new green lamp; kindle it in the house with the oil of the Olive, and the things which shall be in the house shall be made very green, and it shall seem that green and black fowls do fly.

> If thou wilt make a candle or wick to   73
> be shaked, and walk when it is lightened.

Take the skin of a Wolf, and the skin of a Dog, and make of them both a wick, and kindle it with the oil of Olive, and it shall be moved soon.

> When thou wilt lighten a lantern, for   74
> which he shall fear greatly that seeth it.

Take new white linen cloth, and make of it a wick, and put in the hollowness of it a skin of a Serpent and gross salt and fill it with oil [of] Olive, and give it to any man that thou wilt; as soon as he shall kindle it, he shall tremble and fear greatly.

> A marvellous experience, which maketh men   75
> to go into the fire without hurt; or to bear
> fire or red hot Iron in their hand without
> hurt.

Take the juice of *Bismalva* and the white of an egg, and the seed of an herb called *Psyllium*, also *Pulicaria herba*, and break it unto powder, and make a confection, and mix the juice of Radish with the white of the egg. Anoint thy body or hand with this confection, and let it be dried, and after anoint it again. After that thou may suffer boldly the fire without hurt. But if thou wilt that the thing anointed seem to burn, scatter upon it quick Brimstone well beaten into powder, and it shall seem to

§ 73. For similar use of the principle of antagonism, see p. 76.

§ 74. If 'gross salt' is saltpetre, kindling a mixture of it with olive oil might give some cause for fear.

§ 75. *Bismalva* is hollyhock (*Althaea rosea*). *Psyllium* is *Plantago afra* and *pulicaria* is *Pulicaria dysenterica*; Turner (1548) called them respectively fleawort and fleabane—they were supposed to have a repellent effect upon fleas. Colophony is the resinous residue remaining when turpentine is distilled.

be burned, when the Brimstone shall be kindled, and it shall not hurt him. If thou shalt blow the herb called *Colophonia*, [or] Greek Pitch, beaten very small, upon the flame of the candle which a man holdeth in his hand, it augmenteth marvellously the fire, and lifteth up the flame unto the house roof. That thou may bear fire unhurt, let Lime be dissolved with hot water of Beans, and put thereto a little of red earth of Messina; after, put too a little Great Mallows, or Hollyhock, with which, conjoined or mixed together, anoint the palm of thy hand, and let it dry up, and so may thou bear any fire unhurt.

76   Thou mayest make burning water after this fashion.

Take black, thick, mighty and old wine, and in one quart of it thou shalt temper a little quick Lime and Brimstone, beaten into powder very small, and lees of good wine and common salt, white and gross; after thou shalt put it in a gourd, well clayed, and *de super posito alembico*, thou shalt distil burning water, which thou should keep in a glass.

77   Thou mayest make a Greek Fire after this fashion.

Take quick Brimstone, lees of wine, *Sarcocollam*, *Piculam*, sodden salt, oil of stone, and common oil, make them seethe well, and if any thing be put in it, it is kindled, whether it be Tree or Iron, and is not put out but by piss, vinegar or sand.

78   If thou wilt that every thing cease to be marvelled. Look the sufficient causes of doing, and also of suffering, for if thou look both thou shalt not marvel, for thou shalt see that there is so great aptness in one sufficience of another, that it maketh thee not to marvel. For when thou seest that cold water kindled

§ 76. The alembic was a device by which the alchemists distilled liquids; in this case the result might be alcohol of sufficient concentration to burn.

§ 77. *Sarcocollam* is Persian gum, *piculam* 'a little pitch', and 'oil of stone' crude petroleum, all of which are inflammable.

§ 78. This striking passage illustrates clearly the hint of a more modern 'scientific' attitude to be found occasionally in the text. The recipe referred to

the fire, and putteth it not out, if thou should behold the doing cause, thou would marvel always what were the efficient cause convenient to this thing, but when thou lookest to the matter of that effect, that is because it is Lime and Brimstone, which are very inflammable, so that a very little thing flameth them, thou seest that there is nothing to be marvelled.

Likewise it is a marvel that a thing is not burned by fire, when one of the causes is beholden only, but when the nature of the sufferer or weakness of the doer is looked on, there is no marvel.

If thou wilt make a Carbuncle stone,   79
or a thing shining in the night.

Take very many of the little beasts shining by night, and put them beaten small in a bottle of glass, and close it, and bury it in hot Horses' dung, and let it tarry fifteen days. Afterward thou shalt distil water of them *per alembicum*, which thou shalt put in a vessel of crystal or glass. It giveth so great clearness, that every man may read and write in a dark place, where it is. Some men maketh this water of the gall of a Snail, the gall of the Weasel, of the gall of the Ferret, and of a water Dog; they bury them in dung, and distil water out of them.

Make flying fire after this manner.   80

Take one pound of Brimstone, two pound of coals of Willow or Withy, six pound of stony salt; these three things must be brayed very small, in a marble stone. Afterward thou mayest

in the first part of this explanation is on p. 104; see also the note on p. 95. The second paragraph refers to the many recipes which prevent burning, discussed in a note on p. 89.

§ 79. The alembic, again, is an instrument used for distillation. This recipe may result from a confusion with the instructions for a kind of 'invisible ink' described above, p. 96. The 'water Dog' is the otter, *Lutra lutra*.

§ 80. These are accurate instructions for making gunpowder, if the 'salt' is

put some at thy pleasure in a coat of paper, flying or making thunder.

A coat to fly should be long, small and full of that best powder, but a coat to make thunder should be short, gross and half full.

An end of the secrets of nature set forth by
Albertus Magnus in Latin,
newly translated into English.

Imprinted at London, by me
William Copland.

saltpetre (*salis petrosi* in the Latin text). Correct proportions are given, the necessity for very fine grinding in a mortar is clearly stated, and a long, narrow, tightly packed tube would serve as a rocket, while a short, fat, half-filled one would serve as a 'thunder-flash'. Only the information on how to fuse the fireworks is omitted.

LIST OF WORKS CITED IN
THE NOTES TO THE TEXT

Since many of these works use an alphabetical arrangement of subject-matter, page numbers have been indicated only where there might otherwise be confusion.

Aelian (Aelianus, Claudius). *On the Characteristics of Animals*, trans. A. F. Schofield. Loeb Classical Library. 3 vols. London, 1958.

Albertus Magnus. *Opera Omnia*, ed. Augusti Borgnet. 38 vols. Paris, 1890–9.

——. *Book of Minerals*, trans. Dorothy Wyckoff. Oxford, 1967.

Culpeper, Nicholas. *The English Physitian Enlarged*. London, 1669.

Elyot, Sir Thomas. *Bibliotheca Eliotae*. London, 1545 (colophon has 1542). [A Latin dictionary.]

——. *The Castel of Helth*. London, 1537.

Gerard, John. *The Herball, or Generall Historie of Plantes*. London, 1597.

Hortus Sanitatis. An Early English Version of the Hortus Sanitatis, ed. Noel Hudson. London, 1954.

Isidore of Seville. *Etymologiarum sive originum*, ed. W. M. Lindsay. 2 vols. London, 1911.

Kiranides (Cyranus, King of Persia). *The Magic of Kirani King of Persia, and of Harpocration*. London, 1685.

Lupton, Thomas. *A Thousand Notable Things of Sundry Sorts*. London, ? 1579.

Marcus Grecus. *The Book of Fires*, in vol. i (pp. 85–135) of Pierre E. M. Berthelot's *La Chimie au moyen âge*. Paris, 1893.

Pliny (Plinius Secundus, Caius). *Natural History*, trans. H. Rackham *et al.* Loeb Classical Library. 10 vols. London, 1949–62.

Stockholm Medical MS. Reprinted in *Anglia*, xviii (1896), 293–331.

Thorndike, Lynn. *History of Magic and Experimental Science*. 2 vols. New York, 1923.

Topsell, Edward, trans. *The History of Four-footed Beasts and Serpents . . . Collected out of the Writings of Conradus Gesner . . .* London, 1658. Ed. Willy Ley. 3 vols. New York, 1967.

Turner, William. *The Names of Herbes in Greke, Latin, Englishe, Duche and Frenche* (1548), reprinted together with *Libellus de re herbaria* (1538), ed. James Britten *et al.* London, 1965.

Wyckoff, Dorothy. See Albertus Magnus, *Book of Minerals*.

COLLATION

iuxta mēphim urbem in Egipto *C1*
Asbestos] Abaston *C1*
Achates] Agathes *C1*
Amandinus W: Esmundus *C1*
Amethystus] Amaristus *C1*
Heliotropium] Elotropia *C1*
Hephaestites] Epistrites *C1*
Chelidonius] Celidonius *C1*
Gagatronica W: Bagates *C1*
Hyaenia] Bena *C1*
Schistos] Istmos *C1*
Kabrates W: Tabrices *C1*
Gerachidem W: Gerattides *C1*
Nicomar W: Nichomai *C1*
Quiritia W: Quirini *C1*
Radaim W: Radianus *C1*
Liparea] Luperius *C1*
Virites W: Vnces *C1*
Chalazia] Gallasia *C1*
Gagates W: Galerites *C1*
Aetites] Echites *C1*
Hephaestites] Tepristites *C1*
Hyacinthus C2: Hiaciuthus *C1*
Samius W: Saunus *C1*

§ 3. *Ophthalmus W*: Ophethalmius *C1*
obtalmicus L: obtelmicus *C1*
§ 4. Onyx *C2*: Onyz *C1*
§ 5. *Peridonius W*: Fetipēdamus *C1*
§ 6. Tortoise] Corcuses *C1*
tenth day of the Moon *W*: x.
Moone *C1*: luna existente decima *L*
The method of divination is this *W*: But there is mouing of the order, because *C1*: Modus autem ordinis *L*: Modus autem divinationis *Albertus Magnus*
§ 7. lunatic *S*: limatyke *C1*
§ 8. *Medius W*: Medora *C1*

§ 10. *Asbestos*] Abaston *C1*
§ 12. *Achates*] Agathes *C1*
it has black veins] hauing blacke vaynes *C1*
§ 14. *Amandinus W*: Esmundus or Asmadus *C1*
§ 15. *Amethystus*] Amaristus *C1*
§ 17. It is said to have this power . . . waning *W*: it hath no vertue but shyning. Prima cum fuerit, accensa, et crescens monoytes in ultima descendente *C1*: non habet virtutem nisi luna [lucens *in more corrupt eds.*] prima cum fuerit . . . *L*
§ 18. putteth *C2*: that putteth *C1*
§ 20. Heliotropium (twice)] Elitropia *C1*
§ 21. *Hephaestites*] Epibretes *C1*: *Epistretes S*
§ 22. pierced with the stone . . . neck *after W*: perced, & hanged about yᵉ necke, with the stone which is called Sinerip *C1*
§ 23. against] Contra *C1*
Chelidonius] Celidon *C1*
§ 24. *Gagatronica W*: Bagates *C1*
§ 25. *Hyaenia*] Bena *C1*
§ 26. *Schistos*] Histmos *C1*
Granada] Garnade *C1*
§ 27. *Kabrates W*: Tabrices *C1*
§ 29. *Gerachidem W*: Garatides *C1*
§ 30. for the burying *C2*: to the buryenge *C1*
§ 31. *Quiritia W*: Quirim *C1*
§ 32. *Radaim W*: Radianus *C1*
Donatides W: Tonatides *C1*
§ 33. *Liparea*] Luperius *C1*
§ 34. *Virites W*: Vnces *C1*
§ 38. *Chalazia*] Gallasia *C1*
§ 39. *Gagates W*: galeritis *C1*

§ 39. *Kakabre W*: Catabres *C1*
§ 41. *Aetites*] Echites *C1*
    moved] named *C1*: movetur *L*
    that the meat *C2*: the that
    meate *C1*
§ 42. *Hephaestites*] Tepistites *C1*
§ 46. vertigo] a vyrgyn *C1*: verti
    ginem *L*
    Samius W: Saunus *C1*
    Samos *W*: Sauna *C1*
§ 47. Minerals] Mines *C1*: minera
    lium *L*
§ 49. strangury] strangulion *C1*

BOOK III

§ 1. *Tasso L*: Casso *C*: so § 3
§ 13. *Bori*] Boridicta *C1*: Bori dicta
    L
§ 14. If her *S*: If *C1*
§ 20. mastery] a lordship *C1*: possi
    dere vel [sic] dominium et
    virtutem *L*

OF THE PLANETS

    Heading. A short discourse . . .
    planets *J2*: *inserted originally
    after* § *6, p. 65*
§ 2. four of the dial] viii of the dyall
    C1
    sixteen hours of the dial] xvii
    houres of the dyall *C1*
Fig. 21. *Heading*. Of the hours . . .
    nights] *Inserted originally after*
    § *5, p. 65*
§ 5. palace *S*: polayse *C1*: palatium
    L
§ 6. And note . . . evil.] *Inserted
    originally after the table*
§ 10. from the eyes] to the eies *J2*

THE MARVELS OF THE WORLD

§ 2. moveth not] moueth *C1*: non
    moveat *L*
§ 5. altogether] and altogether *C1*
§ 6. Man is the end] a man is the
    ende *C1*
    Man is full] that man is full *C1*
    experience] the experience *C1*
§ 9. *Libri Regimenti*] Libro tegimēti
    C1: so § 19
    aspects] sightes *C1*: aspectibus
    L
§ 13. worketh] it worketh *C1*
    in all things] to al things *C1*
§ 14. proved] an experience *C1*:
    experimentum *L*
    extreme] extremitate *C1*: ex
    terminate *S*: exterminata *L*
§ 15. extreme] extermynate *C1*
    to him boldness] to it boldenes
    C1
    it moveth] that it moveth *C1*
    they make . . . a man] & thei
    are like to a man in this *C1*:
    & assimilant sibi in hoc *L*
§ 20. [until it is tested]] And that
    is not proued *C1*: donec ex
    peritur illud *L*
§ 23. *si cranium* of]si Carneum, if *C1*:
    si cranium *L*
§ 24. *Tyriaca L*: ciriaca *C1*
§ 31. Tabariensis *L*: Taberences *C1*
§ 33. Myrtle] myre *C1*: myrte *S*:
    myrti *L*
§ 41. palate *C2*, *S*: palase *C1*
§ 42. it dieth] it dyeth not *C1*
§ 43. fear in] fear of *C1*
§ 44. *Condisum*] Condicim *C1*
§ 46. *Zinzalas*] zauzales *C1*
§ 52. lamps] thrassholdes *C1*: lumi
    naria *L*

§ 57. or Garlic] or oyle *C1*: aut
   aleum *L*
§ 58. but the gate, and let] but let
   yate, and *C1*: but the yate
   [nisi porta *L*], and let *S*
   fire] mylke *C1*: lar *L*
§ 60. *Cervini*] ceriui *C1*
§ 64. affrayeth *S*: fearyeth *C1*
   drop the water . . . upon it]
   drop doune lyke dewe upō
   the water *C1*

§ 67. do thus *C2*: make *C1*
§ 68. to be cast] cast it *C1*
§ 73. shall be in the house shall be *S*:
   shalbe *C1*
§ 75. Messina] Mitiua *C1*: Missina
   L
§ 77. *Sarcocollam, Piculam*] Sarcecel-
   lam picolam *C1*
§ 78. not burned] burned *C1*: non
   comburitur *L*

INDEX

References are to page numbers of both notes and text; lower-case Roman numerals refer to the Introduction, and major entries are indicated by bold type.